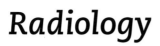

Radiology

To my parents
and to my sister Urmila,
and Ashwinkumar

Radiology

P. R. PATEL

MB, BCh, DMRD, FRCR
Consultant Radiologist
Ealing Hospital, London

Honorary Clinical Senior Lecturer
St Mary's Hospital, London

Blackwell
Science

© 1998 by
Blackwell Science Ltd
Editorial Offices:
Osney Mead, Oxford OX2 0EL
25 John Street, London WC1N 2BL
23 Ainslie Place, Edinburgh EH3 6AJ
350 Main Street, Malden
  MA 02148 5018, USA
54 University Street, Carlton
  Victoria 3053, Australia

Other Editorial Offices:
Blackwell Wissenschafts-Verlag GmbH
Kurfürstendamm 57
10707 Berlin, Germany

Blackwell Science KK
MG Kodenmacho Building
7–10 Kodenmacho Nihombashi
Chuo-ku, Tokyo 104, Japan

First published 1998

Set by Excel Typesetters Co., Hong Kong
Printed and bound in Great Britain
at the University Press, Cambridge

The Blackwell Science logo is a
trade mark of Blackwell Science Ltd,
registered at the United Kingdom
Trade Marks Registry

DISTRIBUTORS

Marston Book Services Ltd
PO Box 269
Abingdon, Oxon OX14 4YN
(Orders: Tel: 01235 465500
         Fax: 01235 465555)

USA
Blackwell Science, Inc.
Commerce Place
350 Main Street
Malden, MA 02148 5018
(Orders: Tel: 800 759 6102
         617 388 8250
         Fax: 617 388 8255)

Canada
Copp Clark Professional
200 Adelaide St West, 3rd Floor
Toronto, Ontario M5H 1W7
(Orders: Tel: 416 597-1616
         800 815-9417
         Fax: 416 597-1617)

Australia
Blackwell Science Pty Ltd
54 University Street
Carlton, Victoria 3053
(Orders: Tel: 3 9347 0300
         Fax: 3 9347 5001)

A catalogue record for this title
is available from the British Library

ISBN 0-632-04758-5

Library of Congress
Cataloging-in-publication Data

Patel, P. R.
    Lecture notes on radiology / P. R. Patel.
        p.   cm.
    Includes bibliographical references
and index.
    ISBN 0-632-04758-5
    1. Radiography, Medical—Outlines,
syllabi, etc. I. Title.
[DNLM. 1. Technology, Radiologic—methods.
2. Diagnostic Imaging—methods.
WN 160 P295L 1997]
RC78.P285 1997
616.07'57—dc21
DNLM/DLC
for Library of Congress   97-10069
                                    CIP

Contents

Preface

This book is intended to be a concise introductory guide to radiology, principally for medical students, but it should also be of value to junior doctors. Additionally, radiographers, many of whom are now involved in procedural and diagnostic methods, may find it beneficial. The contents cover the imaging techniques, basic film interpretation and specialized radiological investigations currently available. Emphasis is on conventional plain film and contrast radiology, as it is essential that interpretation of these fundamentals is mastered before progressing on to more advanced imaging techniques, such as computed tomography (CT) and magnetic resonance imaging (MRI). Despite recent major technological strides, conventional radiology still has a crucial role to play in the assessment of a large number of patients. It is imperative, therefore, that the basics of radiology be learnt, not only to assist patient management, but also because undergraduate examinations tend to focus on these aspects.

Radiology has assumed an important role in the initial diagnosis as well as subsequent management of patients, and I hope that with the introduction of this book it will become a more widely read undergraduate subject. I am well aware, however, of the ever growing burden on the medical curriculum: with this in mind, the format of the book is arranged so that it can be covered easily within a short space of time. The clinical orientation should ensure that the importance of radiology is not taken out of context with the routine care of patients, serving also as an aid to reinforce some essential background information.

The book is divided into sections by body systems, with a brief description of techniques and investigations given at the beginning of several chapters. This should assist understanding of the basic principles of the large number of available procedures for imaging a particular problem, as it is important to be able to choose the correct investigation for each clinical situation. The essentials are presented and discussed in this book in order to provide a basic foundation course in radiology.

P.R.P.

Acknowledgements

I would like to thank all the radiologists, especially Dr R. Eban and Professor P. Lavender, as well as many of my clinician colleagues for their enthusiastic help during the production of this book.

I am particularly grateful to Dr Robert Dick, Consultant Radiologist at the Royal Free Hospital, for his considerable time and effort in scrutinizing most of the manuscript and his helpful suggestions.

The support and encouragement of all the staff at Blackwell Science, including Dr Andrew Robinson, Dr Michael Stein and Catherine Jones has been much appreciated.

Finally I would like to thank my sons, Kinesh and Neil, for their general assistance with the project and their much valued wordprocessing and computer skills.

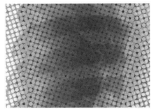

CHAPTER 1

Introduction

INTRODUCTION

Recent technological advances have produced a bewildering array of complex imaging techniques and procedures. The basic principle of imaging, however, remains the anatomical demonstration of a particular region and related abnormalities, the principal imaging modalities being:

- **plain X-rays**: utilizes a collimated X-ray beam to image the chest, abdomen, skeletal structures etc;
- **fluoroscopy**: a continuous X-ray beam produces a moving image to monitor examinations such as barium meals, barium enemas etc;
- **ultrasound (US)**: employs high frequency sound waves to visualize structures in the abdomen, pelvis, neck and peripheral soft tissues;
- **computed tomography (CT)**: obtains cross-sectional computerized densities and images from an X-ray beam/detector system;
- **magnetic resonance imaging (MRI)**; exploits the magnetic properties of hydrogen atoms in the body to produce images;
- **nuclear medicine (NM)**: acquires functional as well as anatomical detail by gamma radiation detection from injected radio-isotopes.

CONTRAST MEDIA

Contrast agents are substances that assist visualization of some structures during the above techniques, working on the basic principle of X-ray absorption, thereby preventing their transmission through the patient. The most commonly used are barium sulphate to outline the gastrointestinal tract, and organic iodine preparations, the latter widely used intravenously in CT for vascular and organ enhancement. Contrast agents can also be introduced into specific sites, for example:

- *arteriography*; the arterial system;
- *venography*: the venous system;
- *myelography*: spinal theca;
- *cholangiography*: the biliary system;
- *hysterosalpingography*: uterus;
- *arthrography*: joints;
- *sialography*: salivary glands.

The possibility of an allergic reaction exists with iodinated contrast media, an increased risk noted in those with a history of allergy, bronchospasm and cardiac disease as well as in the elderly, neonates, diabetics or patients with multiple myeloma.

Minor reactions: Nausea, vomiting, urticarial rash, headache
Intermediate reactions: Hypotension, bronchospasm

Major reactions: Convulsions, pulmonary oedema, cardiac arrhythmias, cardiac arrest.

Drug therapy should be readily available to treat reactions, for example:

urticaria: chlorphenaramine or other antihistamines;

pulmonary oedema: frusemide i.v.;

convulsions: diazepam i.v.;

bronchospasm: hydrocortisone iv and bronchodilators such as salbutamol;

anaphylactic reactions: adrenaline s.c. or i.v.

RADIATION PROTECTION

All individuals receive natural background radiation but diagnostic tests now account for the largest source of exposure and every effort at reduction must be made. Although ionizing radiation is deemed to be potentially hazardous, the risks should be weighed in context of benefits to the patient.

• Doses should be kept to a minimum, a radiological investigation performed only if management is going to be affected. Consideration should be given to the radiation dose to the patient for each specific investigation. CT, barium and radionuclide studies are high dose examinations whereas plain films of the extremities and chest X-rays are typically low dose.

• The fetus is particularly sensitive, especially in the first trimester with possible induction of carcinogenesis or fetal malformation. A menstrual history obtained in a woman of reproductive age, and if necessary a pregnancy test, will prevent accidental fetal exposure to radiation.

• Clear requests to the radiology department, with relevant clinical details aids in the selection of the most appropriate views or investigations.

• Discussion of complex cases with a radiologist may help in choosing the most relevant study or examination.

• Unnecessary examinations should be avoided, for example repeat chest X-rays for resolution of pneumonic consolidation, at less than weekly intervals, or pre-operative chest X-rays in young patients.

• Ultrasound and MRI, because of the lack of ionising radiation, are the preferred imaging modalities where clinically indicated.

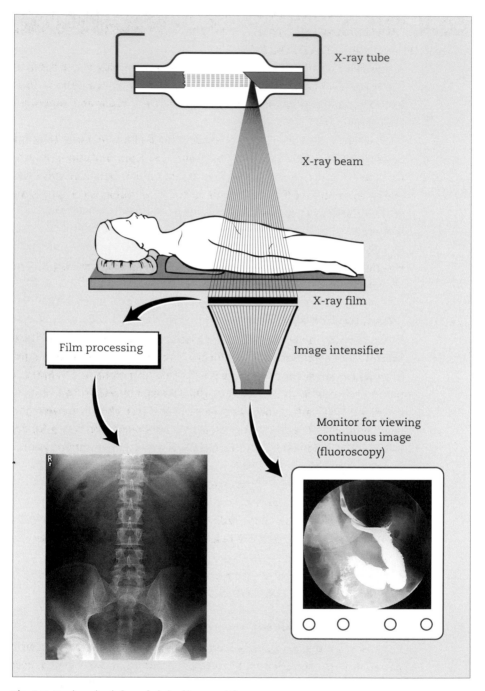

Fig. 1.1 Basic principles of plain films and fluoroscopy.

PLAIN FILMS AND FLUOROSCOPY

CONVENTIONAL RADIOGRAPHY

X-rays are part of the electromagnetic spectrum, emitted as a result of bombardment of a tungsten anode by free electrons from a cathode. Plain films are produced by their passage through the patient and exposing a radiographic film.

Bone absorbs most radiation, causing least film exposure, thus the developed film appears white. Air absorbs least radiation, causing maximum film exposure, so the film appears black. Between these two extremes, a large differential tissue absorption results in a grey scale image. Plain films are particularly useful for:
- chest;
- abdomen;
- skeletal system: trauma, spine, joints, degenerative, metabolic and metastatic disease.

DIGITAL RADIOGRAPHY

In digital radiography, the basic principles are the same but X-ray film is replaced by a digital screen. The information on the screen is then manipulated via computers and the image is visualized on a monitor. CT, MRI and ultrasound are already available in digital format and with introduction of digital plain-film radiography, the long-term goal is to abolish conventional plain films altogether. Some radiological departments are now adopting this new technology (PACS, picture archival and communication system), and although initial investment is large, the principal advantages are:
- significant reduction in radiation exposure;
- digital enhancement ensures all images are of an adequate quality;
- transfer of images out of the radiology department to other sites;
- elimination of storage problems associated with conventional films;
- no missing films;
- rapid retrieval of previous images and reports for comparison;
- ease of availability of examinations to clinicians.

FLUOROSCOPY/SCREENING

Fluoroscopy is the term used when a continuous low-power X-ray beam is passed through the patient to produce a dynamic image that can be viewed on a monitor. Many different procedures, such as barium studies of the gastrointestinal tract, arteriography and interventional precedures are monitored and carried out with the aid of fluoroscopy.

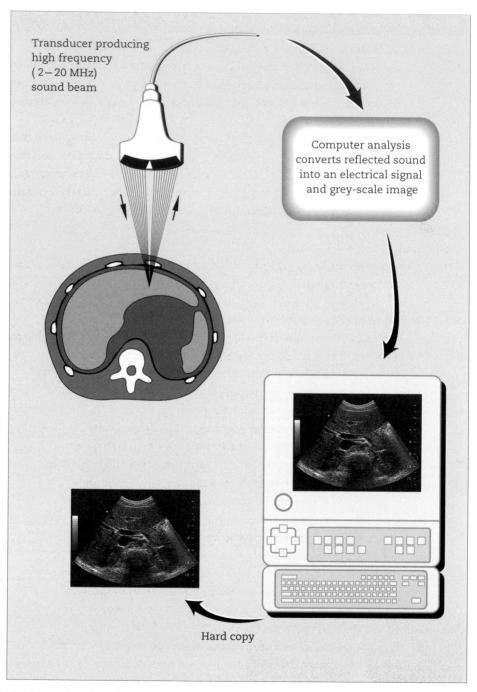

Transducer producing high frequency (2–20 MHz) sound beam

Computer analysis converts reflected sound into an electrical signal and grey-scale image

Hard copy

Fig. 1.2 Basic principles of ultrasound.

ULTRASOUND

Ultrasound employs high-frequency sound waves, produced by a piezo-electric crystal in a transducer. The waves travel through the body, and are reflected back variably, depending on different types of tissues encountered. The same transducer, as well as transmitting ultrasound, receives the reflected sound and converts the signal into an electric current; this is subsequently processed into a grey scale picture. A moving image is obtained as the transducer is advanced across the body (real-time ultrasound). Sections can be obtained in any plane and viewed on a monitor. Bone and air are poor conductors of sound, thus there may be inadequate visualization, whereas fluid has excellent transmission properties.

DOPPLER ULTRASOUND

Doppler ultrasound is a technique to examine moving structures in the body. Blood flow velocities are measured using the principle of a shift in reflected sound frequency produced from moving structures. Utilized for:
- assessment of cardiac chambers and heart valves;
- arterial flow studies, especially carotids and peripheral vascular disease;
- venous flow studies for detection of deep-vein thrombosis.

Uses

Brain: Imaging the neonatal brain.
Thorax: Confirms pleural effusions and pleural masses.
Abdomen: Visualizes liver, gallbladder, pancreas, kidneys etc.
Pelvis: Useful for monitoring pregnancy; uterus and ovaries.
Peripheral: Assesses thyroid, testes and soft-tissue lesions.

Advantages

- Relatively low cost of equipment.
- Non-ionizing and safe.
- Scanning in any plane.
- Can be repeated frequently, for example pregnancy follow up.
- Detection of blood flow, cardiac and fetal movement.
- Portable equipment can be taken to the bedside for ill patients.
- Aids biopsy and drainage procedures.

Disadvantages

- Operator dependent.
- Inability of sound to cross an interface with either gas or bone causes unsatisfactory visualization of underlying structures.
- Scattering of sound through fat produces poor images in obesity.

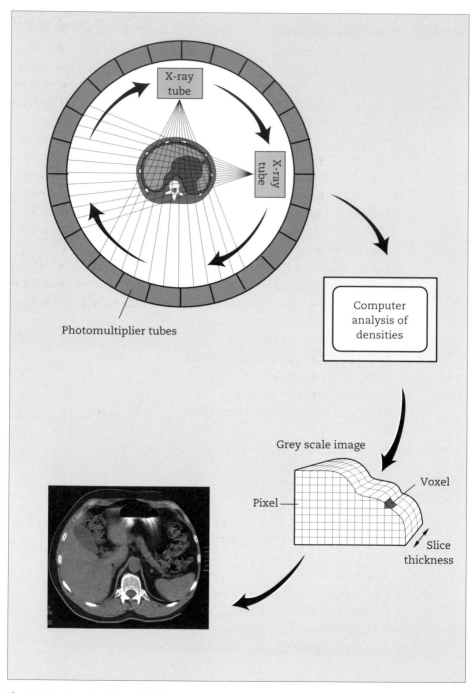

Fig. 1.3 Basic principles of CT.

COMPUTED TOMOGRAPHY

Computed tomography involves passage of a collimated X-ray beam through the patient to obtain images of thin transverse sections of the head and body. Instead of the beam exposing an X-ray film, a more sensitive detection system with photomultiplier tubes is employed. The X-ray tube rotates around the patient during each cycle. An image is obtained by computer processing of the digital readings from the photomultiplier tubes and analysis of the absorption pattern of each tissue. Absorption values are expressed on a scale of $+1000$ units for bone, the maximum absorption of the X-ray beam, to -1000 units for air, the least absorbent.

Each picture represents a section through the body, the thickness being varied from 1 to 10 mm. Tissues lying above or below this slice are not imaged and a series of slices is taken to cover a particular region.

The CT image consists of a matrix of picture elements (pixels), the slice thickness giving the volume component (voxel). Each voxel represents the attenuation value of the X-ray beam at that particular point in the body.

Uses

- Any region of the body can be scanned.
- Staging tumours for secondary spread.
- Radiotherapy planning.
- Exact anatomical detail when ultrasound is not successful.

Advantages

- Good contrast resolution.
- Precise anatomical detail.
- Rapid examination technique.
- In contrast to ultrasound, diagnostic images are obtained in obese patients as fat separates the abdominal organs.

Disadvantages

- High cost of equipment and scan.
- Bone artefacts in brain scanning.
- Scanning mostly restricted to the transverse plane.
- High dose of ionizing radiation for each examination.

SPIRAL (HELICAL) SCANNING

In conventional CT, sections are taken individually with a delay between each one, whereas spiral scanning involves a continuous gradual movement of the patient through the scanner tunnel. The principal advantages are much faster scanning times and improved vascular visualization.

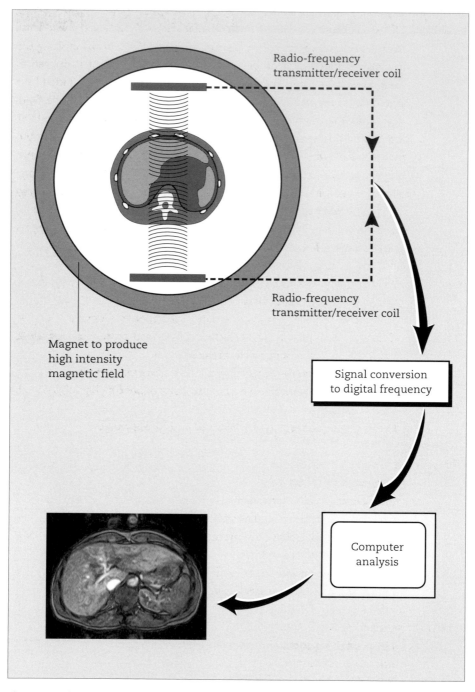

Fig. 1.4 Basic principles of MRI.

MAGNETIC RESONANCE IMAGING

Magnetic resonance scanning produces images of the body by utilizing the magnetic properties of certain nuclei, principally those of hydrogen in water molecules. The patient lies in the scanner tunnel surrounded by a large circular magnet and is subjected to a high-intensity magnetic field. This forces the hydrogen atom nuclei to align with the magnetic field. A pulse of radio-frequency applied to these nuclei then displaces them from their position; when the pulse ceases, they return to their original state, releasing energy (in the form of a radio-frequency signal). Computer analysis processes this energy into a digital signal, with conversion to a grey scale image. Hence, the basic principle of MRI is a study of the response of magnetized tissue to a pulse of radio-frequency, whereby pathological tissue returns different signals compared to normal.

Uses

- CNS: technique of choice for brain and spinal imaging.
- Musculoskeletal: imaging joints and muscular abnormalities.
- Cardiac: imaging with gating techniques related to the cardiac cycle enables the diagnosis of many cardiac conditions.
- Thorax: assessment of vascular structures in the mediastinum.
- Abdomen: structures are well visualized, surrounded by high signal from surrounding fat.
- Pelvis: staging of prostate, bladder and pelvic neoplasms.

Advantages

- Can image in any plane.
- Non-ionizing and hence believed to be safe to use.
- Excellent anatomical detail especially of soft tissues.
- Visualizes blood vessels without contrast: magnetic resonance angiography (MRA).
- No bony artefacts due to lack of signal from bone.
- Intravenous contrast utilized much less frequently than CT.

Disadvantages

- High operating costs.
- Poor images of lung fields.
- Inability to show calcification.
- Fresh blood in recent haemorrhage not as well visualized as by CT.
- MRI more difficult to tolerate with examination times longer than CT.
- Contraindicated in patients with pacemakers, metallic foreign bodies in the eye and arterial aneurysmal clips (may be forced out of position).

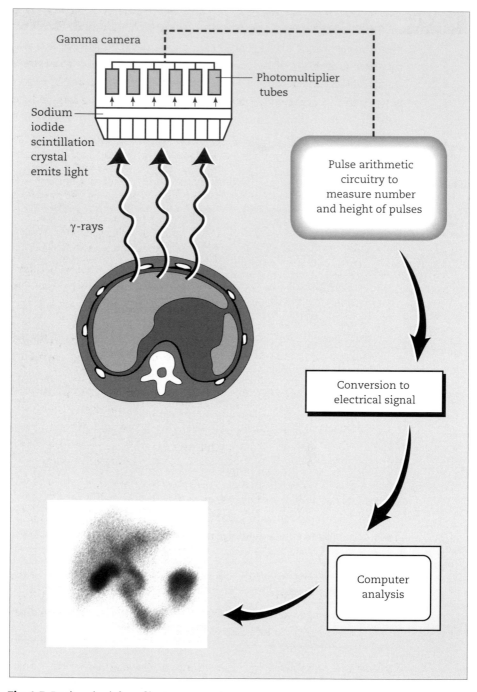

Fig. 1.5 Basic principles of isotope scanning.

NUCLEAR MEDICINE

Radionuclide imaging is a valuable diagnostic tool; the principal modality that examines abnormal physiology of the body in preference to anatomical detail. Technetium-99 m is the commonest isotope used, and by tagging with certain substances a particular region of interest can be targeted.

Anatomical area	Agent	Application
Respiratory tract	99mTc microspheres Krypton, xenon	Perfusion and ventilation scanning for diagnosis of pulmonary embolus
Cardiovascular	Thallium-201	For infarct imaging as it accumulates in normal myocardium showing a defect corresponding to infarcts
Gastrointestinal	Na pertechnetate and 99mTc-labelled WBCs	Studies to detect Meckel's diverticulum and inflammatory bowel conditions
Liver and spleen	Tc-labelled sulphur colloid	Reticuloendothelial uptake to image focal abnormalities
Biliary system	99mTc HIDA	Useful in cholecystitis and obstruction, as isotope uptake in liver is excreted in bile
Urinary tract	DMSA DTPA MAG3	Studies of renal functional and anatomical abnormalities
Skeletal	Tc-labelled phosphonates	Uptake at sites of increased bone turnover, e.g. tumours and arthritis
Thyroid	Iodine-131 or 99 mTc	Assessing focal nodules
Parathyroid	Thallium-201	May visualize adenomas

Table 1.1 Typical applications of isotopes.

SPECT (single-photon emission computed tomography). A planar tomographic 'slice' is reconstructed from photons emitted by the radioisotope. This can be compared with CT 'slices' showing anatomy and shows distribution of radionuclide more clearly.

PET (positron emission tomography). Uses positron-emitting isotopes, many short-lived and cyclotron produced. These agents include radioactive oxygen, carbon and nitrogen. Main clinical applications are in the brain (infarcts and dementia), heart (infarction and angina) and tumours. Accurate studies of blood flow and metabolism are possible using these tracers.

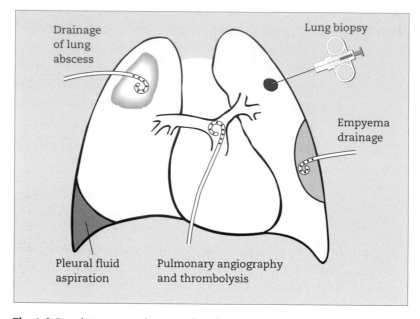

Fig. 1.6 Respiratory tract interventional procedures.

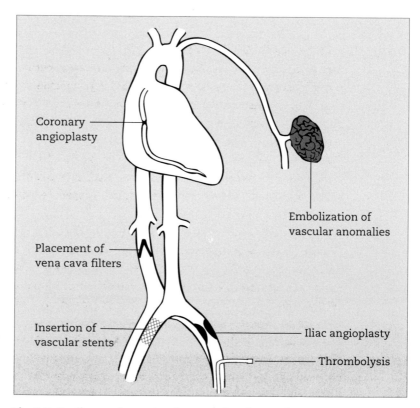

Fig. 1.7 Cardiovascular system interventional procedures.

INTERVENTIONAL RADIOLOGY

RESPIRATORY TRACT

Lung biopsy. A needle is inserted directly into the lung or pleural mass and tissue taken for microbiological or histological analysis. The procedure may be performed under fluoroscopy or CT guidance.

Abscess drainage. A catheter is introduced percutaneously into a lung abscess to achieve drainage.

Pleural fluid aspiration. Ultrasound is effective in diagnosing pleural fluid. Even small quantities can be visualized and aspirated for analysis.

Empyema drainage. Purulent fluid in the pleural cavity, usually due to infection from adjacent structures, can be drained directly by catheter insertion.

Pulmonary angiography. Contrast is injected, via a catheter in the pulmonary artery for the diagnosis of pulmonary embolus. The catheter can be left *in situ* and thrombolytics infused to dissolve blood clot.

CARDIOVASCULAR SYSTEM

Angioplasty. Stenoses in the aorta, iliacs, femorals, peripheral vessels, carotids, coronary vessels, renals and virtually any other artery can be dilated by means of balloon inflation. Narrowed arterial segments and occlusions can also be treated by insertion of metallic stents.

Thrombolysis. Recent arterial thrombus can be lysed by positioning a catheter in the thrombus and infusing streptokinase or TPA (tissue plasminogen activator). Contraindications to this procedure include bleeding diatheses and recent cerebral infarction.

Embolization. The deliberate occlusion of arteries or veins for therapeutic purposes. Steel coils, detachable balloons or various other occluding agents are injected directly into the feeding vessels. Indications include arterial bleeding, arteriovenous fistulae and angiomatous malformations.

Vena cava filter insertion. A filter is introduced percutaneously either through the femoral or internal jugular vein and positioned in the inferior vena cava, just below the renal veins, thus preventing further embolization from thrombus originating in pelvic or lower-limb veins.

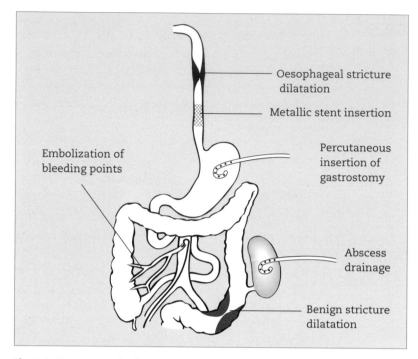

Fig. 1.8 Gastrointestinal tract interventional procedures.

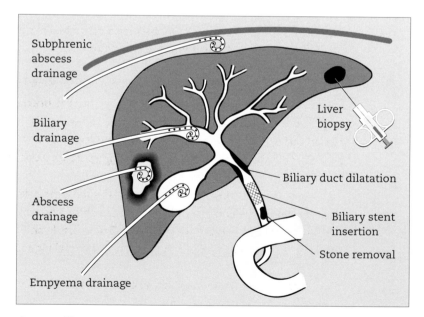

Fig. 1.9 Biliary tract interventional procedures.

GASTROINTESTINAL TRACT

Oesophageal dilatation. A large-diameter balloon is used for dilatation of benign strictures, postoperative anastomotic strictures (e.g. gastro-enterostomy), achalasia and palliation of malignant strictures.

Oesophageal stent. A metallic self-expanding stent is inserted for palliation of malignant oesophageal strictures.

Colonic stricture dilatation. Benign colon strictures, usually anastomotic ones, can be effectively treated by balloon dilatation.

Percutaneous gastrostomy. After gastric distension with air a catheter is inserted directly through the anterior abdominal wall into the stomach.

Embolization. Angiography may localize the bleeding point in severe gastrointestinal haemorrhage. Control of haemorrhage may be possible by infusion of vasopressin or embolization.

Abscess drainage. Percutaneous drainage of subphrenic and pancreatic collections.

BILIARY TRACT

External biliary drainage. In biliary obstruction, a catheter is inserted percutaneously through the liver into the bile ducts.

Internal biliary drainage with endoprosthesis. A plastic or metal stent is positioned within the biliary stricture and free internal drainage achieved without the need for any external catheters. The procedure is preferably carried out by endoscopic retrograde cholangiopancreatography (ERCP), but if this fails, the stent can be inserted using a percutaneous approach.

Biliary stone removal. Postoperatively, when a T-tube is in position and a calculus remains in the common bile duct, a steerable catheter with a basket can be introduced directly through the T-tube track and the calculus extracted. Removal by an ERCP is also an effective technique.

Biliary duct dilatation: balloon dilatation of benign biliary stricture; *liver/subphrenic abscess drainage*; *liver biopsy*.

URINARY TRACT

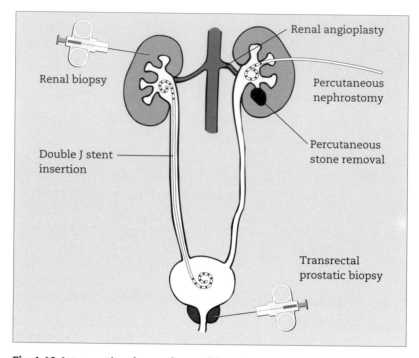

Fig. 1.10 Interventional procedures of the urinary tract.

Renal angioplasty. Balloon dilatation of renal artery stenosis or insertion of metallic stents to alleviate the stenosis (treatment of hypertension or to preserve renal function).

Percutaneous nephrostomy. Insertion of a catheter into the pelvicalyceal system to establish free drainage of urine, when the kidney is obstructed.

Ureteric stent. A special catheter positioned so one end lies in the renal pelvis and the other in the bladder, for the relief of obstruction. Introduction is either from the lower ureter after cystoscopy by a urologist or from above percutaneously under radiological control.

Percutaneous stone removal. Removal of a renal calculus, through a percutaneous track from the posterior abdominal wall directly into the kidney.

Embolization of A-V fistulae. A valuable technique of treating fistulae by introduction of steel coils or other occluding agents into the feeding vessels.

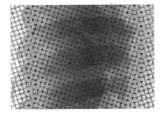

CHAPTER 2

Respiratory Tract

RESPIRATORY TRACT INVESTIGATIONS

PLAIN FILMS

The standard view used is the posteroanterior (PA) projection; others are listed below.

- Anteroposterior (AP): used for ill patients.
- Lateral: localizes an abnormality seen on PA view.
- Supine: valuable in infants and ill patients.
- Oblique: useful to demonstrate pleural, chest wall and rib abnormalities.
- Erect: detects gas under the diaphragm.
- Expiratory: a pneumothorax becomes more prominent.
- Lateral decubitus: small pleural effusions or subpulmonary effusions are recognized more easily with the affected side dependent.

COMPUTED TOMOGRAPHY (CT)

- Excellent detail for staging mediastinal and bronchial neoplasms.
- Valuable in detection of diffuse pulmonary disease.
- Earlier identification of pleural plaques in asbestos exposure.
- Diagnosis of aneurysm or dissection.
- Elucidating the nature of a lung opacity.
- As an aid to lung biopsy.

MAGNETIC RESONANCE IMAGING (MRI)

The principal indications are evaluation of mediastinal masses, aortic dissection and staging bronchial carcinoma, if vascular invasion is suspected.

ULTRASOUND

Ultrasound examination of the chest determines the presence of pleural effusions and loculated fluid. It will accurately locate small quantities of fluid for aspiration. Biopsy of pleural lesions may be carried out using ultrasound guidance.

LUNG BIOPSY

A needle is inserted directly into the mass to be biopsied, obtaining tissue samples. Biopsy should not be carried out if there is a suspicion of an arteriovenous malformation or hydatid cyst. Poor respiratory function is also a contraindication, as a pneumothorax following biopsy may seriously compromise the patient.

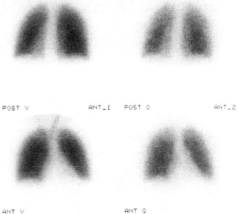

POST V   ANT_1   POST Q   ANT_2

Fig. 2.1 Normal ventilation (V) and perfusion (Q) scan.

ANT V   ANT Q

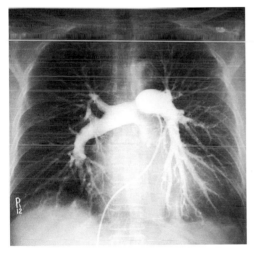

Fig. 2.2 Normal pulmonary angiogram.

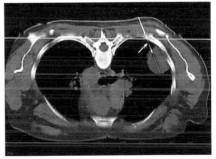

Fig. 2.3 Lung biopsy under CT control. The needle (arrow) has been inserted through the posterior chest wall.

PULMONARY ANGIOGRAPHY

The pulmonary artery is selectively catheterized and contrast injected to visualize the pulmonary arterial and venous circulation.

ISOTOPES

Combined perfusion scanning with technetium-99m-labelled macroaggregates of human albumin and ventilation scanning with inhaled radioactive gas or aerosol typically produces a perfusion defect and not a ventilation defect in pulmonary embolus.

NORMAL CHEST

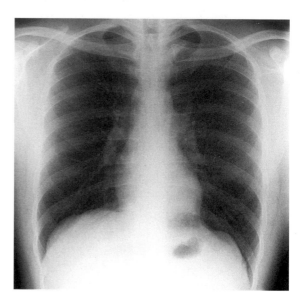

Fig. 2.4 Normal chest X-ray.

Some pertinent radiological considerations

Hilar shadows. Predominantly due to pulmonary arteries: the left hilum is smaller and a little higher than the right.

Horizontal fissure. A white 'hair-line' shadow dividing the right upper and middle lobes and extending up to the right hilum: it is not always seen.

Cardiac shadow. The right atrium is seen just to the right of the thoracic spine. The inferior border is formed by the right ventricle and the left border by the left ventricle.

Diaphragm. The right leaf is usually higher than the left, though occasionally the converse may be true.

Trachea. Lies in the midline with bifurcation at the level of T6. It deviates slightly to the right at the level of the aortic knuckle.

Lung fields. The intrapulmonary arteries radiate from the pulmonary hila and taper towards the periphery contributing to the majority of the lung markings, with a smaller component from the pulmonary veins. The right lung is divided into three lobes: the upper, a small middle lobe and lower lobe. The left lung has two lobes, the upper (including the lingula) and lower.

VIEWING A CHEST FILM

Inspect the film for adequate penetration (lower thoracic spine just visible), inspiration (diaphragms at level of fifth or sixth ribs anteriorly) and rotation (the spinous processes of the upper thoracic vertebrae lie midway between the medial ends of the clavicles).

Examine the chest X-ray systematically to ensure that all areas are covered; skeletal and soft tissues are best left to the end. Keep to a routine but with practice it will be possible to spot the abnormalities and describe them first: lungs; hilar shadows; cardiac shadow; mediastinum; diaphragms; skeletal and soft tissues.

Lungs. Scan both lungs, starting at the apices and working downwards. Compare the appearances of each zone with the other side. (The lungs can be divided approximately into three zones: the upper, middle and lower zones.) The only shadows normally visible, apart from the fissures, should be vascular in origin, so concentrate on searching for any areas of homogeneous shadowing or a mass lesion. It may be easier to describe an opacity within a zone and later determine the lung lobe.

Hilar shadows. A common site for lymphadenopathy and bronchial carcinoma: look for increased density and irregularity as well as enlargement of the hilar shadow.

Cardiac shadow. Note the size and shape. Specific chamber enlargement is often difficult to identify: pay attention to and comment on the overall size of the heart.

Mediastinum. Assess for mass lesions and also for mediastinal shift by position of the trachea and cardiac shadow.

Diaphragms. The costophrenic angles should be clear, sharp and deep. Blunting may indicate a pleural effusion or old pleural thickening. The upper surfaces should be clearly defined: poor definition often implies basal lung pathology. Flattening of the diaphragms suggests hyperinflation and chronic obstructive airways disease.

Skeletal and soft tissues. Look at the periphery of the film; ribs for fractures or secondary deposits; appearances of the breast shadows and whether there has been a mastectomy; under diaphragms; shoulders etc.

PRINCIPAL TYPES OF LUNG SHADOWING

NORMAL APPEARANCES

The lungs appear translucent with only branches of the pulmonary arteries and veins visible. There is no other shadowing.

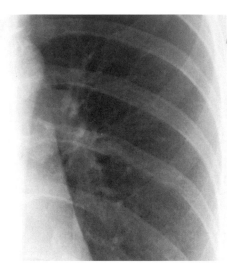

Fig. 2.5 Normal lung fields.

RETICULAR/INTERSTITIAL SHADOWING

This is produced by thickening of the tissues around the alveoli, the lung interstitium, and visualized as a fine or coarse branching linear pattern. Typical conditions giving rise to this type of shadowing are lung fibrosis and pneumoconiosis.

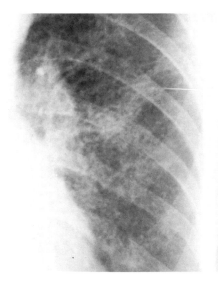

Fig. 2.6 Interstitial lung shadowing.

NODULAR SHADOWING

Nodular shadowing is due to small discrete spherical opacities 1–5 mm in diameter. Causes include: miliary tuberculosis; pneumoconiosis; sarcoidosis; neoplastic: miliary carcinomatosis from thyroid, melanoma, etc.

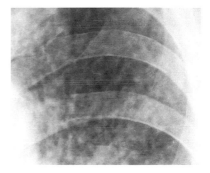

Fig. 2.7 Nodular shadowing.

CONSOLIDATION

Consolidation is due to replacement of air in the alveoli by fluid or occasionally tissue, resulting in areas of confluent homogeneous shadowing. Patent bronchi and some small airways are often still visible as linear lucencies, when surrounded by fluid-filled alveoli: this sign is called an air bronchogram.

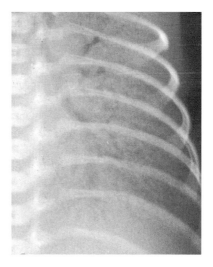

Fig. 2.8 Consolidation showing an air bronchogram.

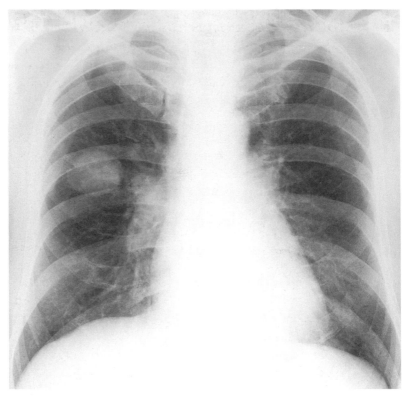

Fig. 2.9 Bronchial carcinoma: solitary circular opacity in the right mid-zone ('coin lesion').

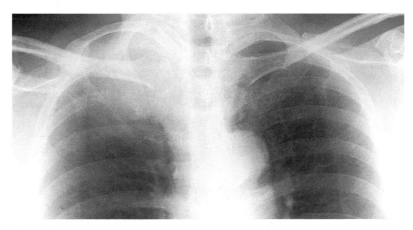

Fig. 2.10 Pancoast's tumour: mass at the right apex with rib destruction.

BRONCHIAL CARCINOMA: PERIPHERAL

This is a common primary tumour, with approximately half found in the peripheral lung fields. The main histological types are squamous, small (oat) cell, anaplastic, adenocarcinoma and the rarer alveolar cell carcinoma.

PRESENTATION

Haemoptysis; respiratory symptoms such as cough and shortness of breath; weight loss; cerebral or lymph-node metastases; slowly resolving pneumonia; routine chest; paraneoplastic syndromes such as inappropriate antidiuretic hormone (ADH) secretion.

RADIOLOGICAL FEATURES

Bronchoscopy may be negative in peripheral lesions, as visualization is not possible distal to the segmental bronchi. The following features may be present on a plain chest film.
- Lobulated or spiculated mass but sometimes with a smooth outline.
- Associated hilar gland enlargement, pleural effusion, areas of collapse or consolidation.
- Cavitation found in 15% with central air lucency, an air/fluid level and a wall of variable thickness. Squamous carcinomas frequently cavitate.
- Tumours at the lung apex (Pancoast's tumour) can invade the brachial plexus, resulting in shoulder and arm pain with wasting of the hand, or invasion of the sympathetic chain may give rise to Horner's syndrome.

Further investigations include:
- *CT/MRI chest and upper abdomen.* Assesses spread and determines operability. This examination will establish whether there has been any metastatic spread into the mediastinal lymph nodes, chest wall, liver or adrenals. MRI is generally more accurate in defining mediastinal and vascular invasion.
- *Lung biopsy.* Either under fluoroscopy or CT control to obtain a sample for histology.

DIFFERENTIAL DIAGNOSIS OF SOLITARY LUNG MASS

- Metastasis: sometimes single, most commonly from breast, kidney, colon and testicular tumours.
- Tuberculoma: often apical and may have areas of calcification.
- Benign neoplasms: bronchial adenoma (usually perihilar), hamartoma (most common benign tumour of the lung), rarely focal areas of pneumonia, hydatid cyst, haematoma or arteriovenous malformation.

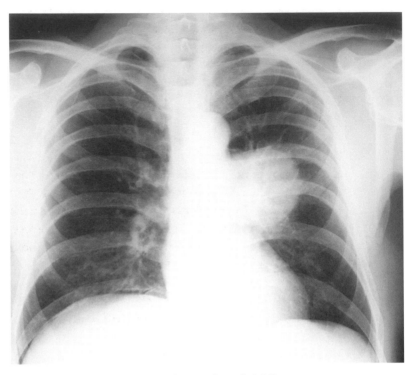

Fig. 2.11 Central bronchial carcinoma: large left hilar mass.

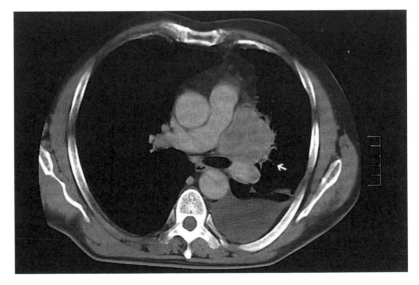

Fig. 2.12 CT scan demonstrating the left hilar mass (arrow). There is no associated lymphadenopathy but a left pleural effusion is present.

BRONCHIAL CARCINOMA: CENTRAL

Central bronchial carcinoma arises from the major bronchi, causing a mass in the hilar region.

PRESENTATION

As in peripheral carcinoma.

RADIOLOGICAL FEATURES

On a *chest X-ray*, the central mass causes the hilar shadow to enlarge, assume an increased density or an irregular outline. As the tumour increases in size, narrowing of the bronchial lumen may cause collapse of the distal lung and consolidation due to secondary infection. A large tumour often gives rise to complete collapse of a lung and may result in opacification of the entire hemithorax.

CT/MRI aids identification of extent and spread of the tumour to:
* lymph nodes: mediastinal and hilar lymphadenopathy;
* oesophagus: direct invasion with dysphagia or fistula;
* pleura: pleural effusion;
* pericardium: pericardial effusion;
* bone: direct extension into sternum or ribs;
* superior vena cava: obstruction with venous engorgement.

Common sites of distant metastases are:
* brain;
* bone;
* adrenals;
* liver.

Lymphangitis carcinomatosa: dissemination of carcinoma through lymphatic channels of the lung, usually unilateral, but may be bilateral.

Invasion of the tumour may also involve the phrenic nerve (elevation of the diaphragm) or laryngeal nerve (hoarseness).

TREATMENT

* Surgical resection: inoperable if direct invasion or distant metastases.
* Chemotherapy: especially for oat cell carcinoma.
* Radiotherapy: inoperable tumours or when complications arise:
   brain metastases;
   spinal cord compression;
   superior vena cava obstruction.

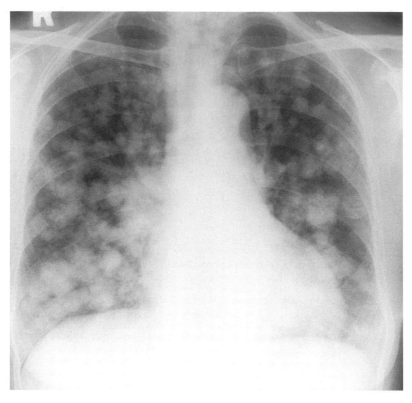

Fig. 2.13 Widespread pulmonary metastases.

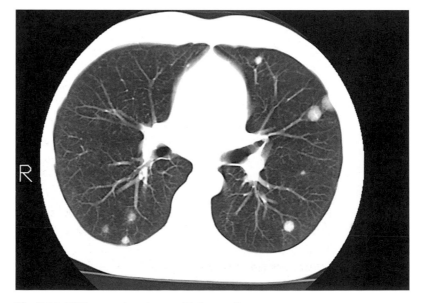

Fig. 2.14 CT thorax showing multiple small metastases.

PULMONARY METASTASES

Metastatic disease to the lungs and rib cage is a common complication of primary neoplastic disease originating elsewhere, usually through the haematogenous route. Tumours of the breast, renal tract, testis, gastrointestinal tract, thyroid and bone are often the primary source.

RADIOLOGICAL FEATURES

Abnormalities can be seen on either plain films or CT. Metastatic disease to the chest may involve one or more of the following: lungs; pleura; lymph nodes; local invasion; bony skeleton.

Lungs

Virtually any malignancy may give secondary deposits in the lungs. Deposits usually appear as well-defined, multiple, round opacities of differing sizes in the lung fields. CT is particularly sensitive in detecting metastases not visible on a chest X-ray and helpful in monitoring response to chemotherapy. Opacities just a few millimetres across can be easily visualized. Cavitation is occasionally present, usually indicating metastases from squamous cell carcinoma.

Pleura

Pleural metastases are often from breast carcinoma, and may be visualized as mass lesions, though the most common manifestation is a pleural effusion, masking the underlying pathology.

Lymph nodes

CT is accurate in the detection of enlarged hilar and mediastinal lymph nodes. (CT will detect nodes 1 cm in size and smaller, but nodes <1 cm are less likely to be metastatic.)

Lymphangitis carcinomatosa — secondary deposits in central lymph nodes may produce lymphatic congestion with a linear pulmonary pattern radiating outwards from the hilar glands, septal lines and pleural effusions.

Local invasion

Pericardium to give malignant pericardial effusion; superior vena cava compression or obstruction; phrenic nerve paralysis; Pancoast's tumour.

Skeletal system: ribs, thoracic spine, shoulder girdle

Deposits may be lytic, e.g. from breast, sclerotic from prostate, or mixed.

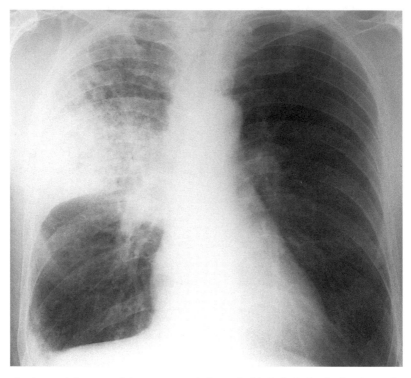

Fig. 2.15 Right upper lobe pneumonia bounded inferiorly by the horizontal fissure. Blunting at the right costophrenic angle is due to a pleural effusion.

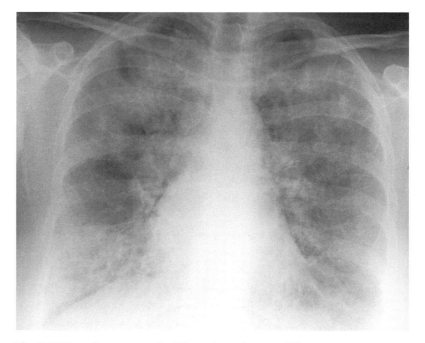

Fig. 2.16 Bronchopneumonia: bilateral patchy consolidation.

PNEUMONIA

Pneumonia, an inflammatory reaction in the lungs, occurs either as a primary infection of the lungs, or secondary to bronchial obstruction.

Primary pneumonia. Inflammation arising in a normal lung.

Secondary pneumonia. Caused by:
- occluded bronchus from bronchial carcinoma or foreign body;
- aspiration from pharyngeal pouch, oesophageal obstruction;
- underlying lung pathology: bronchiectasis, cystic fibrosis.

Lobar pneumonia. Inflammatory changes confined to a lobe, classically due to *Streptococcus pneumoniae*.

Bronchopneumonia. Produces bilateral multifocal areas of consolidation.

RADIOLOGICAL FEATURES

On a plain film, it is generally not possible to diagnose the infecting agent from the type of shadowing. The affected part of lung assumes an increased density with inflammatory exudate and fluid occupying the alveolar space. Air still remaining in the affected bronchi appears as linear lucencies (consolidation with air bronchogram). Consolidation may persist, often after the patient's symptoms have improved. CT is not required for primary pneumonia, but allows assessment of complications.

TYPES OF PNEUMONIA

- Viral pneumonia: most common pneumonia in children.
- *Streptococcal* pneumonia: commonest cause of bacterial pneumonia.
- *Mycoplasma* pneumonia (primary atypical pneumonia): commonest cause of non-bacterial pneumonia, often with slow resolution.
- *Staphylococcal* pneumonia: most frequent cause of bronchopneumonia and secondary invader in influenza.
- *Klebsiella* pneumonia: predominantly seen in elderly, debilitated patients.
- *Legionella* pneumonia: a rapidly progressive pneumonia, often in the lower lobes and associated with systemic involvement affecting other organs, especially the liver and kidneys.
- *Pneumocystis carinii* pneumonia: typically affects patients with acquired immune deficiency syndrome (AIDS) or those who are immunosuppressed; diffuse perihilar changes progress to alveolar consolidation.
- Radiation pneumonia: pneumonic consolidation arising in the field of radiotherapy.

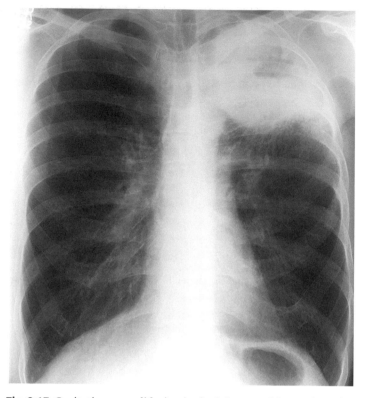

Fig. 2.17 Cavitating consolidation in the left upper lobe: active tuberculosis.

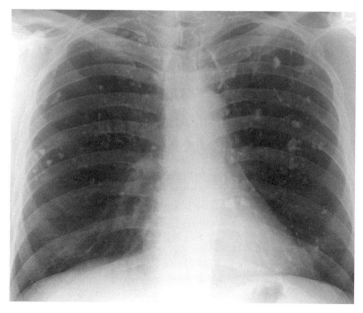

Fig. 2.18 Old healed calcified tuberculous foci.

TUBERCULOSIS

Tuberculosis is a chronic infection caused by *Mycobacterium tuberculosis*, affecting mainly the respiratory tract, though it can involve any system in the body. The immigrant population, debilitated or immunosuppressed patients are all prone to the infection.

RADIOLOGICAL FEATURES

In *primary tuberculosis* the following may be present on a chest X-ray:

• Area of peripheral pneumonic consolidation (Ghon focus) with enlarged hilar mediastinal glands (primary complex). This usually heals with calcification.

• Areas of consolidation which may be small, lobar or more extensive throughout the lung fields.

Postprimary tuberculosis or reactive tuberculosis:

• Patchy consolidation, especially in the upper lobes or apical segments of the lower lobes, often with cavitation.

• Pleural effusions, empyema or pleural thickening.

• Miliary tuberculosis: discrete 1–2 mm nodules distributed evenly throughout the lung fields due to haematogenous spread.

• Mediastinal or hilar lymphadenopathy is not a feature, except in acquired immune deficiency syndrome (AIDS) patients.

As healing progresses, features that may be recognized are: fibrosis and volume loss; calcified foci; tuberculoma: a localized granuloma often containing calcification; pleural calcification.

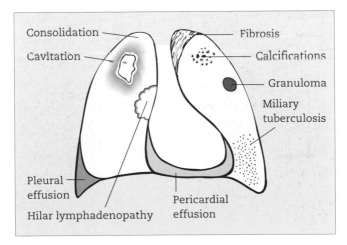

Fig. 2.19 Manifestations of pulmonary tuberculosis.

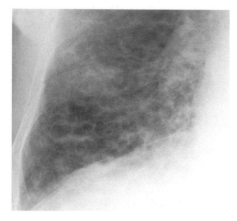

Fig. 2.20 Cystic bronchiectasis: ring opacities at the right base.

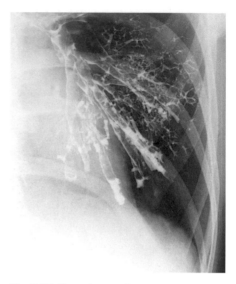

Fig. 2.21 Bronchography: now an obsolete technique but elegantly demonstrates cylindrical bronchiectasis with dilatation of the lower lobe bronchi.

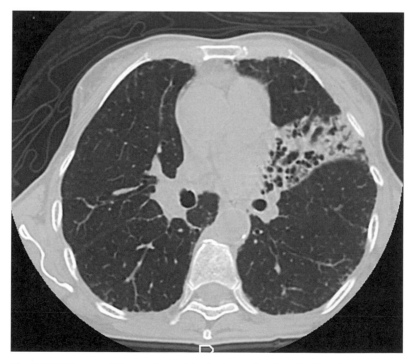

Fig. 2.22 CT scan of thorax: bronchiectasis confined to the lingula.

BRONCHIECTASIS

Bronchiectasis is defined as a condition in which there is an irreversible dilatation of the bronchi. The main aetiological factors appear to be obstruction leading to distal bronchial dilatation and infection causing permanent bronchial wall damage.

PRESENTATION

Cough with purulent sputum; haemoptysis; recurrent chest infections.

RADIOLOGICAL FEATURES

The chest film may be entirely normal. Bronchiectasis is commonest at the lung bases and a chest X-ray may reveal the following features.
• *Cylindrical bronchiectasis*: dilated bronchi may be visible as parallel lines (representing the bronchial walls) radiating from the hilum towards the diaphragm
• *Cystic bronchiectasis*: terminal dilatation may be visualized as cystic or ring shadows, sometimes with fluid levels.
• Pneumonic consolidation.
• Fibrotic changes.

High-resolution CT unequivocally demonstrates bronchial dilatation and thickened bronchial walls. It can also define which lobes are affected, especially important to identify if surgery is needed. On CT, the following additional features may be observed:
• bronchi visible peripherally;
• bronchus larger in diameter than the adjacent pulmonary artery branch.

COMPLICATIONS

Empyema; cerebral abscess; amyloid.

CAUSES

Childhood infections: following measles and whooping cough complicated by pneumonia.
Aspergillosis: hypersensitivity reaction in the bronchial walls in asthmatics resulting in bronchiectasis which affects proximal airways.
Bronchial obstruction: foreign body, neoplasm or tuberculosis.
Cystic fibrosis: viscid sputum leading to bronchial obstruction and bronchiectasis.
Congenital: Kartagener's syndrome (dextrocardia, sinusitis and bronchiectasis).

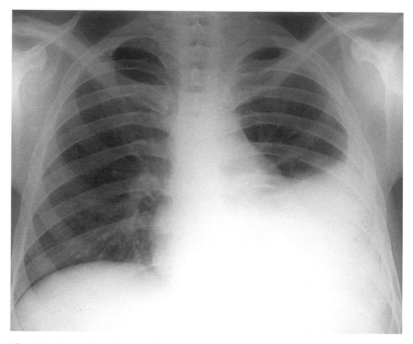

Fig. 2.23 Large left pleural effusion.

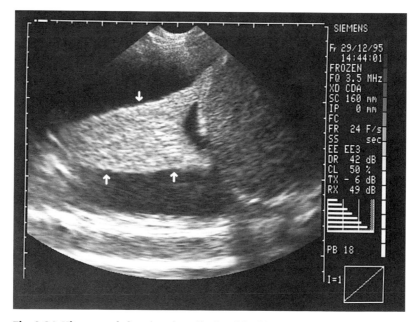

Fig. 2.24 Ultrasound showing the effusion (black) surrounding the retracted lung (arrows).

PLEURAL EFFUSION

Pleural effusion, a fluid collection in the space between the parietal and visceral layers of the pleura, usually contains serous fluid, but may have differing contents.

Haemothorax:	Blood, usually following trauma.
Empyema:	Purulent fluid from extension of pneumonia or lung abscess.
Chylothorax:	Chyle from rupture of the thoracic duct or secondary to malignant invasion.
Hydropneumothorax:	Fluid and air.

RADIOLOGICAL INVESTIGATIONS

Chest film; Ultrasound; CT.

RADIOLOGICAL APPEARANCES

Pleural fluid, in the erect position, gravitates to the lower-most part of the thorax with the following features on a chest X-ray:
- homogeneous opacification, generally of the same density as the cardiac shadow;
- loss of the diaphragm outline;
- no visible pulmonary or bronchial markings;
- concave upper border with the highest level in the axilla.

As the fluid collection grows in size, the underlying lung decreases in volume and retracts towards the hilum. Initially the fluid accumulates in the posterior, then the lateral costophrenic space. When fluid is detected on a standard PA chest film, by blunting of the costophrenic angle, the pleural effusion will already contain 200–300 ml. With larger effusions, there is a mediastinal shift to the opposite side.

Subpulmonary effusion. Caused by fluid accumulating between the diaphragm and the inferior part of the lung. The upper margin of the shadow of the fluid runs parallel to the diaphragm and on the PA chest film mimics a high diaphragm.

Loculated effusion. Fluid can loculate in the fissures or against the chest wall, and this is occasionally seen in cardiac failure.
- Ultrasound is a highly sensitive examination in detecting pleural fluid.
- CT may also demonstrate pleural effusions and visualize underlying abnormalities.

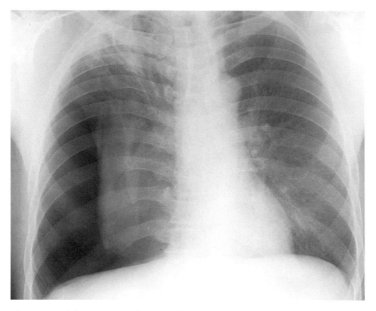

Fig. 2.25 Right pneumothorax: there are no visible markings beyond the lung edge.

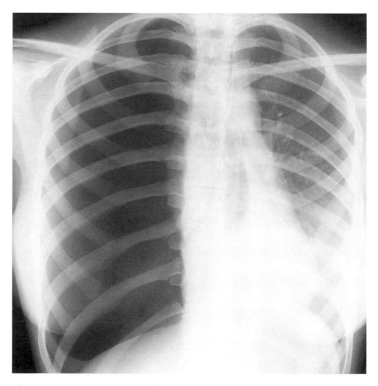

Fig. 2.26 Tension pneumothorax with complete collapse of the right lung and mediastinal shift to the left.

PNEUMOTHORAX

A pneumothorax occurs when air enters the pleural cavity by a tear in either the parietal or visceral pleura; the lung subsequently relaxes and retracts to a varying extent towards the hilum. Small pneumothoraces are difficult to diagnose and usually become more prominent on expiratory films.

RADIOLOGICAL FEATURES

Pneumothorax is best demonstrated on an underpenetrated chest film. The following may be seen.

- Lung edge: a thin white line of the lung margin, the visceral pleura.
- Absent lung markings between the lung edge and chest wall.
- Mediastinal shift: when a tension pneumothorax develops.

CAUSES

- Iatrogenic (one of the commonest causes): following lung biopsy, chest aspiration, thoracic surgery and central line insertion.
- Spontaneous: most common in tall, thin, young males; usually due to rupture of a small pleural bleb.
- Trauma: stab wounds, rib fractures. Surgical emphysema is commonly associated with air tracking along the muscle planes of the chest wall.
- Pre-existing lung disease: increased incidence of pneumothorax with underlying lung disease such as emphysema, cystic fibrosis or interstitial lung disease.

COMPLICATIONS

- Tension pneumothorax: a tear in the visceral pleura may act as a ball valve allowing air to enter the pleural cavity during each inspiration, and none to escape during expiration. Positive pressure builds up, resulting in a dramatic shift of the mediastinum away from the side of the pneumothorax. This is a medical emergency, as death can rapidly ensue from respiratory distress and diminished cardiac output.
- Hydropneumothorax: fluid in a pneumothorax.

TREATMENT

Generally, a small pneumothorax with less than 20% collapse of the lung requires no treatment. Pleural air will reabsorb with subsequent lung expansion. Larger pneumothoraces can be treated by aspiration or insertion of a chest drain with an underwater seal. Follow-up films are required to ensure complete resolution of the pneumothorax.

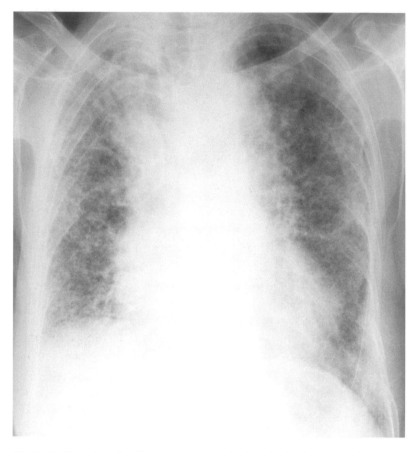

Fig. 2.27 Fibrosing alveolitis: extensive reticular shadowing throughout both lungs.

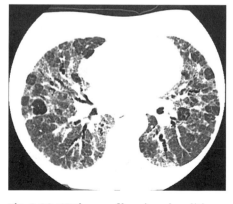

Fig. 2.28 CT thorax: fibrosing alveolitis with coarse linear fibrotic strands.

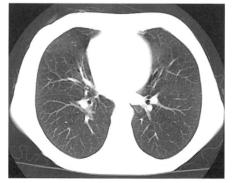

Fig. 2.29 Normal CT thorax at the same level.

FIBROSING ALVEOLITIS

Fibrosing alveolitis is a disease of unknown aetiology, but probably auto-immune, in which an inflammatory reaction in the alveolar wall leads to pulmonary fibrosis. It is more common in males, and in the 40–70 age group. Prognosis is poor with a greater than 50% mortality over 5 years.

PRESENTATION

Progressive dyspnoea; cough; clubbing.

RADIOLOGICAL FEATURES

In early disease, the chest X-ray may be normal, but as fibrosis progresses the following features may exist.

• Fine nodular and streaky linear shadowing (reticulonodular pattern) starting at the bases but may involve all the lung fields.

• Honeycomb pattern in severe disease, with small cystic spaces and coarse reticulonodular shadowing.

• Reduction in lung volume.

• Poor definition of the cardiac outline due to adjacent lung fibrosis.

• Dilatation of pulmonary arteries with right ventricular enlargement and pulmonary hypertension.

High-resolution CT sections define lung parenchymal changes earlier and the examination is more precise than a chest X-ray. CT is effective in monitoring progress of the disease.

CAUSES OF LUNG FIBROSIS

• Sarcoidosis.
• Cystic fibrosis.
• Pneumoconiosis.
• Rheumatoid lung.
• Systemic sclerosis.
• Drugs: nitrofurantoin, cyclophosphamide.

COMPLICATIONS

• Pneumothorax.
• Cor pulmonale.

TREATMENT

• Steroids.
• Immunosuppressive therapy.

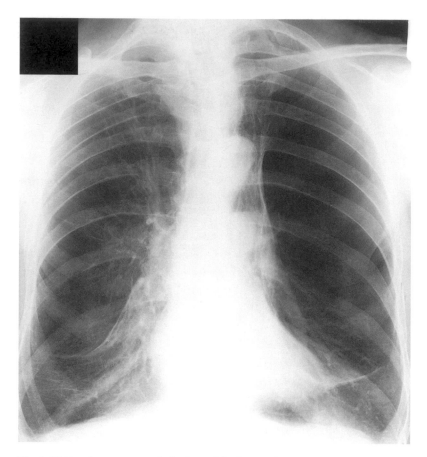

Fig. 2.30 Emphysema: overinflation of the lungs, flattened diaphragms, bullae and a small cardiac shadow.

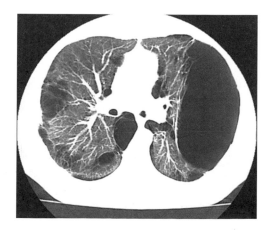

Fig. 2.31 CT thorax: multiple destructive areas resulting in bullae of varying sizes.

EMPHYSEMA

Emphysema is a condition in which there is an increase in the size of the air spaces, with dilatation and destruction of lung tissue distal to the terminal bronchiole. Cigarette smokers and coal miners have a higher incidence, and rarely there may be an association with α_1-antitrypsin deficiency (in which emphysema predominantly affects the lower lobes).

RADIOLOGICAL FEATURES

The chest X-ray may be entirely normal despite severe debility of the patient. In advanced emphysema the following may be found.

Hyperinflation of the chest

• Low flat diaphragms with limited excursion in inspiration and expiration.
• Increase in the AP diameter of the chest with an expansion in the retrosternal clear space (barrel chest)
• Thin, long and narrow appearance to the heart shadow, likely to be from overinflation and low diaphragms, rather than an actual change in heart size.

Vascular changes

• The lungs are generally unevenly affected with an abnormal distribution of pulmonary vasculature; blood vessels are attenuated, with loss of the normal smooth gradation of vessels from the hilum to the periphery.
• Pulmonary hypertension leading to cor pulmonale. The proximal pulmonary arteries progressively enlarge and right-heart failure develops.

Bullae

Cyst-like spaces often develop from rupture of distended alveoli. On a chest film, they are seen as translucent areas with their walls shown as thin curvilinear hair-line shadows. They vary in size from a few centimetres in diameter to occupying a large part of the hemithorax, displacing and compressing adjacent normal lung.

TERMINOLOGY

The term 'emphysema' is also used in:
• *Mediastinal emphysema*: air within tissue planes of the mediastinum.
• *Surgical emphysema*: air tracking along the soft-tissue planes; in the chest, this may be found after thoracic surgery or a pneumothorax.
• *Obstructive emphysema*: a bronchus partially occluded by a mass or foreign body causing a ball valve obstruction.

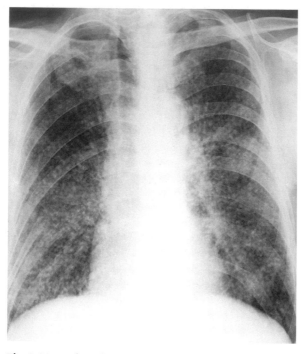

Fig. 2.32 Coal worker's pneumoconiosis: coarse nodular shadowing.

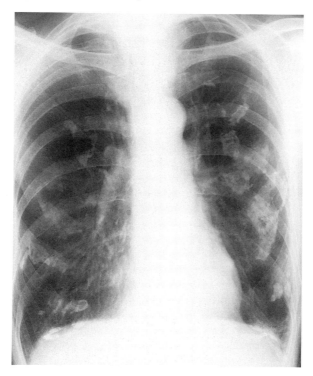

Fig. 2.33 Calcified pleural plaques in asbestos exposure.

PNEUMOCONIOSIS

Pneumoconiosis is a condition caused by the inhalation of dust into the lungs. A history of dust exposure is present.

RADIOLOGICAL APPEARANCES

Appearances depend on whether the dust is active or inactive.

Active dust: Silica and coal dust are potent producers of diffuse lung fibrosis, although in the early stages small lung nodules are a characteristic feature.

Inactive dust: Iron oxide, calcium compounds and barium produce a fine nodular pattern, due to deposits of dust particles.

Organic dust: Exposure can also cause lung fibrosis examples being:
- Bird-fancier's lung: pigeon and budgerigar excreta;
- Farmer's lung: mouldy hay;
- Bagassosis: sugar-cane dust.

COMPLICATIONS

- Progressive massive fibrosis.
- Caplan's syndrome.
- Emphysema.
- Cor pulmonale.

ASBESTOS EXPOSURE

RADIOLOGICAL APPEARANCES

With previous exposure to asbestos, the following may be seen on a chest X-ray:
- Focal pleural plaques: often the earliest finding, seen lying adjacent to ribs.
- Calcified pleural plaques: bilateral diaphragmatic calcifications are very suggestive of previous asbestos contact.
- Diffuse pleural thickening.
- Pleural effusions: often bilateral.
- Pulmonary fibrosis, especially basal though the whole lung, may be involved leading to cor pulmonale. Reticular shadowing commences at the bases and may obscure the sharp outline of the heart border.
- Malignant disease. There is a much higher incidence of:
  mesothelioma (chest and peritoneal);
  bronchial carcinoma, laryngeal carcinoma.

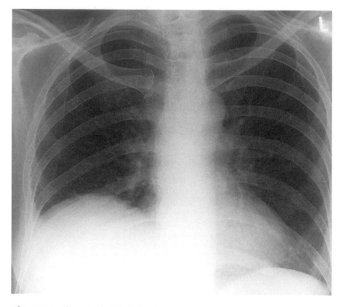

Fig. 2.34 Elevated right diaphragm.

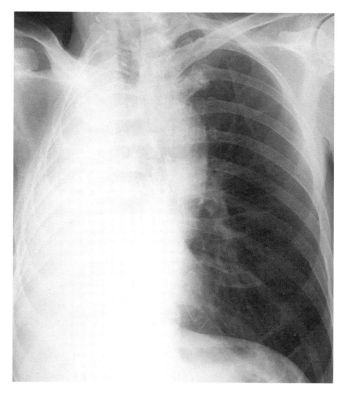

Fig. 2.35 Complete opacification of the right hemithorax: collapse of the right lung with significant mediastinal shift to the right (note position of the trachea and cardiac shadow).

ELEVATED DIAPHRAGM

The diaphragm consists of a thin sheet of muscle with a smooth upward convexity, the right usually lying in a higher position than the left. On a chest film, the inferior surface of the diaphragm is not visualized as it blends with the surfaces of the liver and spleen.

CAUSES OF A UNILATERAL ELEVATED DIAPHRAGM

- Above diaphragm: phrenic nerve palsy; infiltration from bronchial carcinoma or mediastinal tumour.
- Diaphragm: eventration, more common on the left and results from deficiency or atrophy of muscle.
- Below diaphragm: right diaphragm elevation; liver or subphrenic abscess, liver secondary deposits.

CAUSES OF BILATERAL ELEVATED DIAPHRAGMS

- Obesity.
- Hepatosplenomegaly.
- Within the abdomen: ascites, pregnancy, abdominal masses.

OPAQUE HEMITHORAX

Complete opacification of a hemithorax is encountered in the following conditions. (Mediastinal shift is assessed by the position of the trachea and the heart.)

With mediastinal shift away from opaque hemithorax: pleural effusion; large pleural effusions may occupy the whole of the hemithorax.

With mediastinum central: consolidation; in severe pneumonia, consolidation may render the whole lung opaque.

With mediastinal shift towards opaque hemithorax:

- Lung collapse: most commonly occurs from total occlusion of a main bronchus either by a central bronchial carcinoma or a postoperative mucus plug. The lung collapses and is devoid of air, hence the appearance of a dense hemithorax.
- Post pneumonectomy: after resection of a lung, the empty hemithorax fills with fluid. Gradual reabsorption with a fibrotic reaction eventually results in opacification with a significant mediastinal shift towards the pneumonectomy.

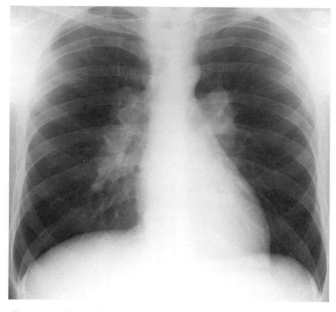

Fig. 2.36 Bilateral hilar lymphadenopathy.

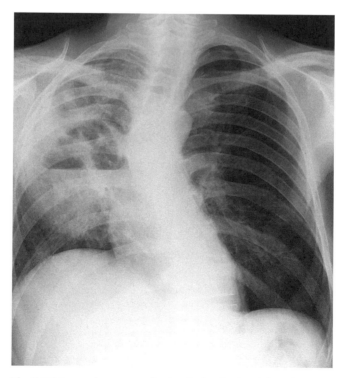

Fig. 2.37 Lung abscess: cavitating lesion in the right mid-zone with a fluid level.

HILAR LYMPHADENOPATHY

Hilar lymphadenopathy may cause enlargement of the hilar shadows, the lymph nodes appearing as well-defined, lobulated masses. Nodal enlargement has to be differentiated from hilar vascular prominence (as in pulmonary hypertension). Difficulty may be encountered in distinguishing between them on chest radiography, though CT with contrast or MRI accurately identifies the abnormality.

CAUSES OF BILATERAL HILAR GLAND ENLARGEMENT
- Sarcoidosis: commonest cause, usually resolving spontaneously.
- Lymphoma: mediastinal glands are more frequently involved than hilar.
- Tuberculosis: enlargement is usually asymmetrical and often associated with mediastinal glandular involvement.
- Metastases.

CAUSES OF UNILATERAL HILAR GLAND ENLARGEMENT
- Bronchial carcinoma.
- Lymphoma.
- Tuberculosis.

LUNG ABSCESS

A lung abscess is a localized necrotic, cavitating lesion due to a pyogenic infection. Secondary abscess formation may occur from aspiration under anaesthesia, inhalation of vomit or foreign body, oesophageal disease such as achalasia and carcinoma of the oesophagus or septic material aspiration from upper-airway passages.

RADIOLOGICAL FEATURES
Abscess formation may initially start as an area of pneumonic consolidation (especially *Staphylococcus aureus* or *Klebsiella pneumoniae*) with subsequent development of cavitation. A fluid level is often noted in the abscess.

DIFFERENTIAL DIAGNOSIS OF A CAVITATING LESION
- Carcinoma: primary bronchial carcinoma is the commonest cause; solitary cavitating secondary deposit. A benign cavity has a central cavity and a regular wall whereas a malignant one has an eccentric cavity with an irregular wall.
- Tuberculosis.
- Cavitating pulmonary infarct, haematoma or infected bulla (rare).

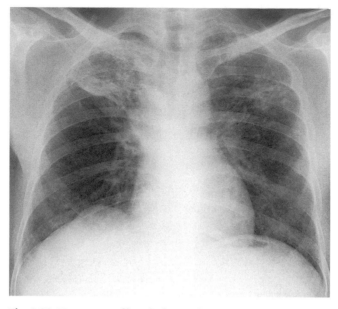

Fig. 2.38 Upper zone fibrosis from tuberculosis.

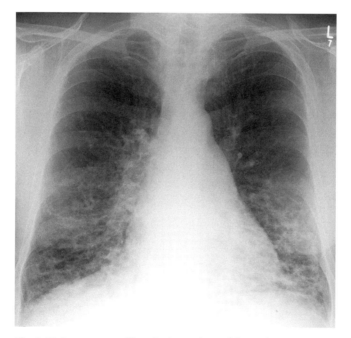

Fig. 2.39 Lower zone fibrosis due to bronchiectasis.

UPPER-ZONE FIBROSIS

Fibrosis may affect predominantly the apices and upper zones, with sparing of the lower zones in the following conditions:

- Tuberculosis: associated with calcified areas and pleural thickening.
- Sarcoidosis: hilar lymphadenopathy may also be present.
- Radiotherapy: usually following treatment for carcinoma of the breast.
- Ankylosing spondylitis: fibrosis usually occurs when the spinal disease is severe.
- Chronic extrinsic allergic alveolitis: hypersensitivity reaction to inhalation of specific antigens, e.g. from pigeons and budgerigars; the chest X-ray is often normal but may show patchy consolidation in the acute stages, but in chronic disease fibrotic shadowing is predominantly in the upper zones.

LOWER-ZONE FIBROSIS

Fibrosis in the lower zones may obscure the heart border and produce a 'shaggy heart' appearance. Fibrosis predominantly affects the lower zones in:

- Bronchiectasis or long-standing infection.
- Cryptogenic fibrosing alveolitis.
- Rheumatoid arthritis.
- Radiotherapy: usually following treatment for carcinoma of the breast.
- Asbestos exposure.
- Scleroderma: an autoimmune disease with fibrosis of interstitial lung tissue, predominantly basal but may involve the whole lung. The disease commonly affects the joints, skin, gut and respiratory tract.

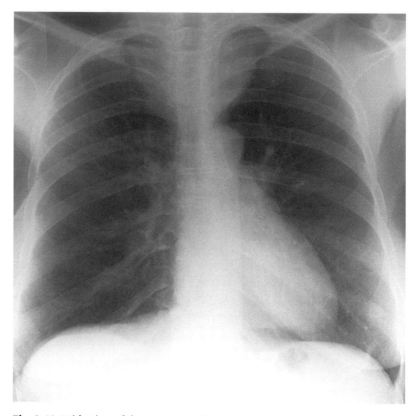

Fig. 2.40 Widening of the upper mediastinum from a retrosternal thyroid.

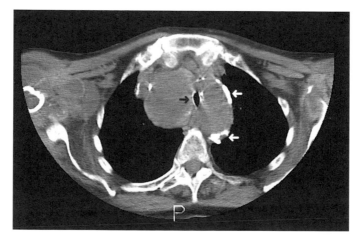

Fig. 2.41 CT upper thorax: retrosternal thyroid causing tracheal narrowing (→). Note calcified areas in the mass (←).

MEDIASTINAL MASS

The mediastinum is that part of the chest bounded by the sternum at the front, thoracic spine at the back and laterally by the medial surfaces of visceral pleura. It can be divided into: anterior mediastinum: anterior to the pericardium; middle mediastinum: the heart, aortic root and pulmonary vessels; posterior mediastinum: behind the posterior pericardial surface.

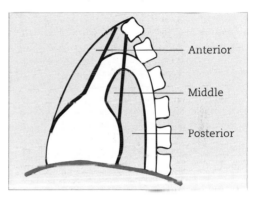

Anterior

Middle

Posterior

Fig. 2.42 Mediastinal compartments.

Although the mediastinum is categorized into compartments, masses may freely cross from one part to another.

RADIOLOGICAL FEATURES

Usually, a mediastinal mass is suspected on a plain chest film; a lateral film may be helpful; further evaluation is carried out by CT/MRI for anatomical localization. The presence of cystic lesions, calcification, fat and vascular structures are all more accurately assessed than by plain films.

• *Anterior mediastinal masses (three Ts—thyroid, thymus and teratodermoids)*
Retrosternal thyroid: the mass is well defined and may be lobulated. Extension into the mediastinum is to a varying degree up to the carina.

Thymic tumours: these may be benign or malignant and frequently associated with myasthenia gravis.

Teratodermoids: these tumours are usually benign but have a malignant potential. Occasionally fat, rim calcification, bone fragments and teeth may be identified.

• *Middle mediastinal masses*
Lymphadenopathy: lymphoma, metastases, sarcoid or tuberculosis.

• *Posterior mediastinal masses*
Neurogenic tumours arising from intercostal nerves and sympathetic chain.

Neurofibromas (nerve sheath tumours).

Ganglioneuroma (sympathetic nerve cell tumours).

RIGHT UPPER-LOBE COLLAPSE

The right upper-lobe collapses with movement of the horizontal fissure upwards, pivoting at the hilum in both the PA and lateral projections. The collapsed lobe assumes an increased density at the right apex, its lower border being sharply defined by the horizontal fissure. The hilum may be elevated.

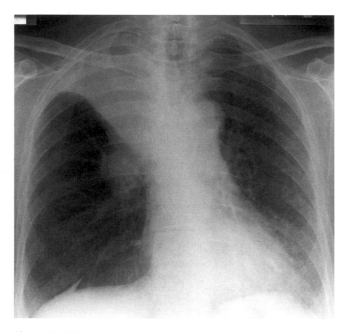

Fig. 2.43 Right upper-lobe collapse due to a mass at the right hilum.

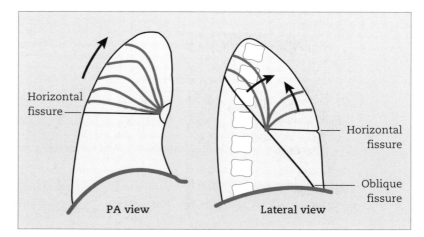

Fig. 2.44 Movement of the fissures in right upper-lobe collapse.

RIGHT MIDDLE-LOBE COLLAPSE

The middle lobe is relatively small. On the PA view, middle-lobe collapse produces only minor changes, with some increased density lateral to the right cardiac border with blurring of the cardiac outline (silhouette sign). It is most accurately evaluated using the lateral projection, where the collapsed lobe is seen as a triangular opacity projected over the cardiac shadow.

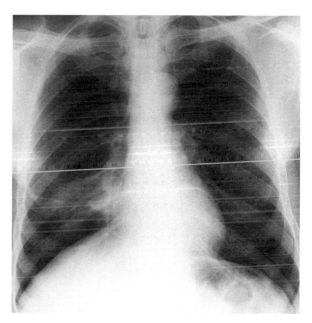

Fig. 2.45 Right middle-lobe collapse. PA view. Note loss of right heart border.

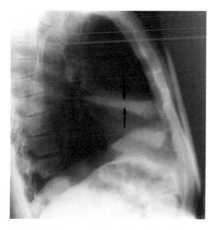

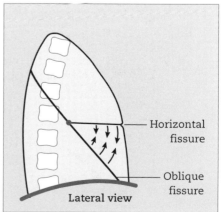

Fig. 2.46 Lateral view showing the collapse projected over the cardiac shadow. (Arrows.)

Fig. 2.47 Movement of fissures in right middle-lobe collapse.

LEFT UPPER-LOBE COLLAPSE

The lobe collapses in a different fashion to the right upper lobe. Movement of the oblique fissure is forwards and the collapsed lobe lies anteriorly against the chest wall, giving rise to a hazy, ill-defined opacity in the upper and mid-zones on the PA projection.

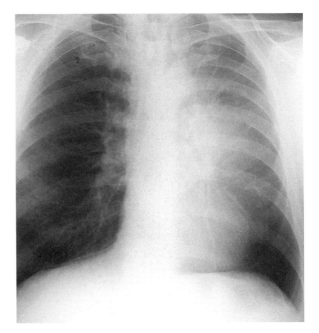

Fig. 2.48 Left upper-lobe collapse with hazy ill-defined shadowing in the left upper and mid-zone.

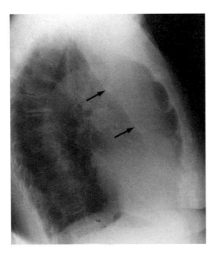

Fig. 2.49 Lateral view shows the lobe collapses anteriorly. (Arrows.)

Fig. 2.50 The oblique fissure moves forwards in left upper-lobe collapse.

Lateral view

RIGHT/LEFT LOWER-LOBE COLLAPSE

The lower lobes collapse medially and posteriorly. The oblique fissure moves backwards maintaining the same slope. On the PA film, left lower-lobe collapse is seen as a triangular area projected through the cardiac shadow.

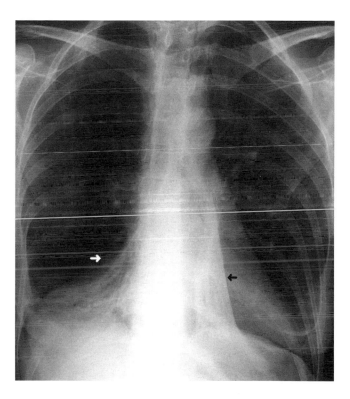

Fig. 2.51 Bilateral lower-lobe collapse (arrows), the left more clearly defined.

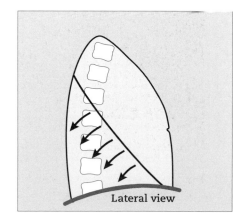

Fig. 2.52 The oblique fissure moves backwards in lower lobe collapse.

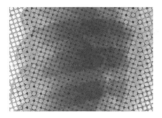

CHAPTER 3

Cardiovascular
System

CARDIOVASCULAR INVESTIGATIONS

PLAIN FILMS

Evaluate heart size and chamber enlargement. On a standard chest projection, the ratio of the cardiac diameter to that of the maximum internal diameter of the chest should be no greater than 50% on a full inspiratory film.

ULTRASOUND

Echocardiography and Doppler examination reveal anatomical abnormalities as well as flow disturbances and assist in the study of incompetent and stenotic valves, aortic arch aneurysms, dissecting aneurysms, cardiomyopathy and pericardial effusions.

ISOTOPE SCANNING

Technetium-99m pyrophosphate accumulates in damaged myocardium whereas thallium-201 produces a deficient uptake in territories supplied by occluded or narrowed arteries. Thallium is most commonly used as a screening technique in patients with suspected coronary artery disease.

COMPUTED TOMOGRAPHY (CT)

Relevant applications include the further evaluation and diagnosis of dissecting thoracic aneurysms, pericardial effusions and myocardial tumours.

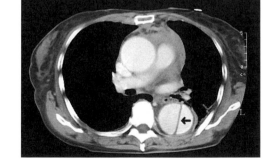

Fig. 3.1 Dissection of the descending aorta. Note the intimal flap in the contrast filled aorta (arrow) and blood in the mediastinum.

MAGNETIC RESONANCE IMAGING (MRI)

MRI can be gated to the cardiac cycle to reduce motion artefact. It can examine the heart in any plane and is of value in many clinical situations including pericardial effusions, hypertrophic cardiomyopathy, and congenital and valvular heart disease. Magnetic resonance angiography (MRA) has the capability of providing a non-invasive method of imaging many vascular abnormalities such as aneurysm, dissection, stenoses, occlusions and congenital anomalies.

ARTERIOGRAPHY

Vascular access is usually obtained using a percutaneous approach via the femoral artery. Any major vessel or blood supply to an organ can be studied by selective arterial cannulation with contrast injection. Radial, brachial, axillary or popliteal arteries can also be punctured percutaneously, if femoral artery access is unsuitable. Anatomical detail is excellent; haematoma, haemorrhage and arterial thrombus are recognized rare local complications.

INTRAVENOUS DIGITAL SUBTRACTION ANGIOGRAPHY

This technique is utilized to visualize the arterial system by injection of a bolus of contrast into the superior vena cava. After passage through the heart and lungs, the dilute contrast may be imaged in the arterial circulation by computer subtraction. Resolution is not as detailed as conventional arteriography, but can be an effective investigation in many clinical situations.

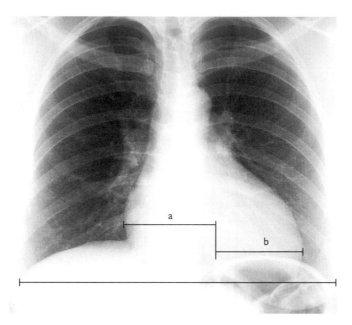

Fig. 3.2 Cardiomegaly the heart size is measured by comparing the cardiac diameter (a+b) to the maximum internal diameter of the chest.

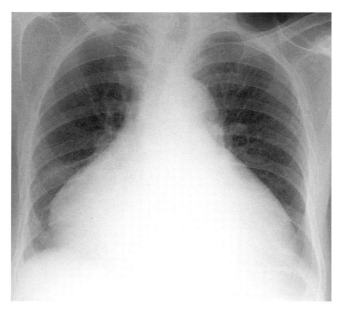

Fig. 3.3 Pericardial effusion: large globular shaped cardiac shadow with clear lung fields.

CARDIOMEGALY

On a standard PA chest, the heart size can be expressed as the cardiothoracic ratio. Generally, a ratio of over 50% of the heart size to the maximum internal diameter of the chest indicates cardiac enlargement. This measurement is only an approximate guide, and is helpful for serial measurement. Specific chamber enlargement is often difficult to identify, but a plain chest film may show the following:

Left atrium: the only chamber that can be reliably diagnosed when it is enlarged; it may feature a double contour to the right heart border, splaying of the carina with upward displacement of the left main bronchus or posterior bulging the chamber on a lateral chest X-ray.

Right atrium: prominence of the right heart border.

Right ventricle: upward displacement of the cardiac apex with anterior enlargement of the heart border on a lateral projection.

Left ventricle: increased convexity of left heart border.

Echocardiography is more accurate in the assessment of specific chamber and cardiac size.

PERICARDIAL EFFUSION

A pericardial effusion is a collection of fluid in the pericardial sac, the fluid being either serous, blood or lymphatic in origin.

RADIOLOGICAL FEATURES

• *Chest film*: illustrates a symmetrically enlarged and globular cardiac shadow only when there is a significant effusion (>250 ml). Pericardial effusion should be suspected if there has been a rapid serial increase in the cardiac shadow, with normal pulmonary vasculature.

• *Echocardiography*: the investigation of choice. Effusions are visible as echo-free areas surrounding the heart.

• CT: may also identify the aetiology, e.g. mediastinal malignancy.

• MRI: accurate for diagnosis and also images the chest and mediastinum.

CAUSES

Infective (viral, bacterial, tuberculous); uraemia; postmyocardial infarction (Dressler's syndrome); myxoedema; malignancy: bronchial and mediastinal tumours with pericardial invasion; collagen vascular diseases (systemic lupus erythematosus (SLE), rheumatoid arthritis).

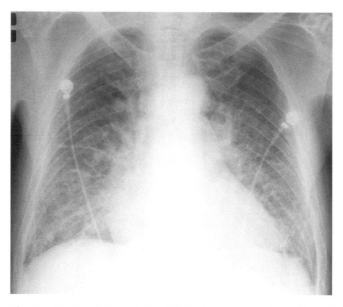

Fig. 3.4 Cardiac failure: interstitial pulmonary oedema. Note fluid in the right horizontal fissure.

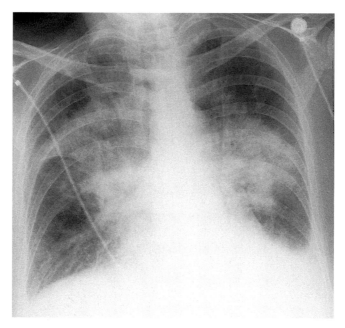

Fig. 3.5 Alveolar pulmonary oedema; fluid accumulating predominantly in the perihilar region; left pleural effusion.

CARDIAC FAILURE

Cardiac failure is said to be present when tissue demands cannot be adequately supplied by the heart. It is usually due to low output from ischaemic heart disease but, paradoxically, may rarely result from high output as a consequence of excessive tissue needs in conditions such as thyrotoxicosis or Paget's disease.

RADIOLOGICAL FEATURES

On a chest X-ray the following may be seen:
• Cardiac enlargement.
• Upper-lobe vascular prominence: from raised pulmonary venous pressure.
• Pleural effusions: seen as blunting at the costophrenic angles, but as the effusions become larger, there is a homogeneous basal opacity with a concave upper border.
• Interstitial pulmonary oedema: initially, prominence of the upper-lobe and narrowing of the lower-lobe vessels. As venous pressure rises, interstitial oedema develops and fluid accumulates in the *interlobular areas* with peripheral septal lines (Kerley 'B' lines).
• Alveolar pulmonary oedema. With further increases in venous pressure, fluid transgresses into the alveolar spaces (alveolar shadowing) with haziness and blurring in the perihilar regions; in severe cases, pulmonary oedema develops throughout both lung fields. The outer thirds of the lungs may be spared, the bilateral central oedema being described as 'bat's wing'.

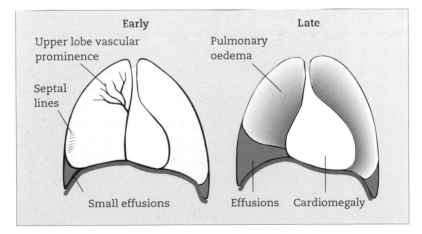

Fig. 3.6 Manifestations of cardiac failure.

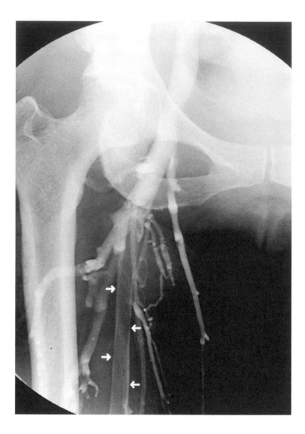

Fig. 3.7 Lower limb venogram: recent thrombus in the femoral vein seen as a filling defect with contrast around the thrombus (arrows). The contrast filled common femoral and iliac vein appear normal.

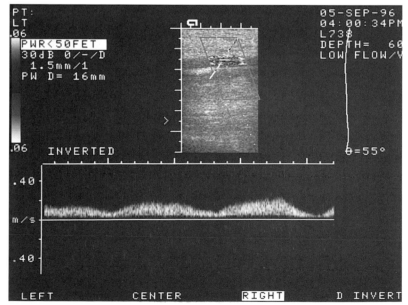

Fig. 3.8 Doppler examination of the femoral vein with a normal Doppler signal and blood flow.

DEEP-VEIN THROMBOSIS

Thrombus formation in the deep veins of the calf is a common clinical problem. Predisposing causes include recent surgery, contraceptive use, prolonged bed rest, neoplastic disease and hypercoaguability states.

PRESENTATION

- Calf swelling.
- Calf pain.
- Pulmonary embolus may be the first sign, the calves being asymptomatic.

RADIOLOGICAL INVESTIGATIONS

- Colour Doppler ultrasound.
- Venography.

RADIOLOGICAL FEATURES

Colour Doppler ultrasound is the initial investigation of choice but difficulty may be encountered in visualizing calf veins especially in obese patients. If there is a strong clinical suspicion, in the presence of a normal Doppler examination, venography is suggested.

- *Colour Doppler ultrasound.* Accurately images vascular flow patterns and the presence of thrombus in the lower limbs. Blood clot may be seen within the vein lumen, often accompanied by a reduction in blood flow.

- *Venography.* Contrast is injected into a foot vein to visualize the lower-limb circulation. Tourniquets applied at the ankle and above the knee force the contrast into the deep veins, thrombus being visualized as filling defects in the vein lumen. Extensive thrombus formation may lead to poor or complete lack of contrast filling of the veins.

COMPLICATIONS

- Pulmonary embolus.
- Postphlebitic syndrome.

TREATMENT

- Heparin.
- Anticoagulants.
- Vena cava filter insertion in recurrent pulmonary embolization. Introduced percutaneously via the femoral or internal jugular vein and positioned in the inferior vena cava, just below the renal veins.

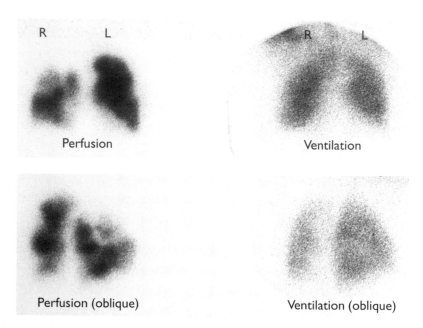

Fig. 3.9 Ventilation and perfusion isotope scans in both the frontal and oblique projections showing mismatched defects suggesting pulmonary emboli.

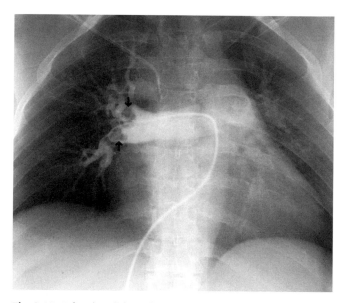

Fig. 3.10 Selective right pulmonary angiogram: thrombus in the right main pulmonary artery (arrows) with poor distal perfusion.

PULMONARY EMBOLUS

Pulmonary embolism occurs when a blood clot detaches from the periph-eral venous system and lodges in the pulmonary artery or its branches.

Pulmonary infarction is the lesion that develops secondary to pulmonary embolus. Predisposing causes include prolonged bed rest, recent surgery, pregnancy, hypercoagulable states and lower limb deep-vein thrombosis.

RADIOLOGICAL FEATURES

The blood clot usually originates from the pelvic or lower-limb veins and migrates into the pulmonary circulation. The chest X-ray is normal in the majority of cases, but if pulmonary infarction develops as a consequence of embolus, any of the following may be seen:

- raised diaphragm;
- small pleural effusions;
- basal collapse or plate-like atelectasis;
- consolidation, often segmental, peripherally situated and wedge shaped.
- *Isotope scan.* Pulmonary embolus results in a segmental defect in perfu-sion with preserved ventilation (ventilation/perfusion mismatch).
- *Pulmonary arteriography.* The definitive examination for the diagnosis of pulmonary embolus and indicated if surgical intervention is to be consid-ered. Arteriography demonstrates blood clot in the pulmonary artery as intraluminal filling defects with obstruction and attenuation of the pul-monary arterial branches. Infusion of thrombolytics through the catheter may lyse the clot. Dynamic spiral CT is equivalent to arteriography in the detection of emboli in the proximal vessels and is a less invasive technique.

COMPLICATIONS

Pulmonary hypertension: resolves in the acute stage when thrombi disin-tegrate. However, it may persist with recurrent embolization.

TYPES OF EMBOLISM

- *Fat embolism.* Usually seen after severe skeletal trauma with fat globules entering the circulation and obstructing pulmonary vessels.
- *Septic embolism.* Arising from tricuspid endocarditis or infected material from central venous pressure (CVP) lines, pacing wires, etc.
- *Amniotic fluid embolism.* Commonest cause of postpartum maternal death. Amniotic debris may gain access to the maternal circulation with subsequent embolization.

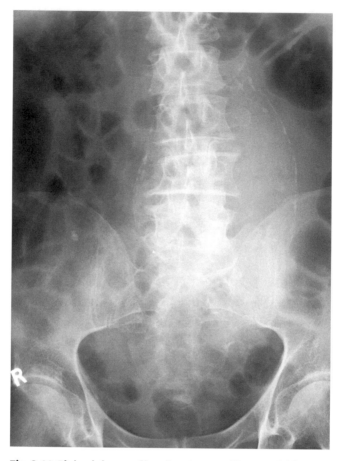

Fig. 3.11 Plain abdomen film showing curvilinear calcification in a large abdominal aortic aneurysm.

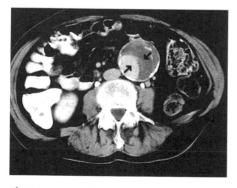

Fig. 3.12 CT abdomen after contrast shows filling of the lumen (↗)and thrombus in an aneurysm (↙).

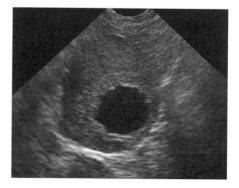

Fig. 3.13 Transverse ultrasound of the abdomen showing the lumen (black) surrounded by thrombus.

ABDOMINAL AORTIC ANEURYSM

An 'aneurysm' refers to a localized dilatation of the vessel wall. Aneurysms may arise in any part of the aorta, but are most frequently seen in the abdominal aorta below the level of the renal arteries. Degenerative vascular disease with subsequent weakening of the vessel wall is the usual cause.

PRESENTATION

Asymptomatic finding; abdominal pain or back pain from vertebral erosion; pulsatile abdominal mass; acute abdomen.

RADIOLOGICAL FEATURES

• *Plain abdominal films* may show curvilinear calcification in the wall of an aneurysm, especially when due to atherosclerosis. Calcification is more clearly visualized on a lateral abdominal film.

• *Ultrasound* is the best initial investigation to determine the presence of an aneurysm, measurement of its diameter and to assess subsequent progress. An increased threat of rupture exists with those > 6 cm in diameter and elective surgery is recommended.

• *CT/MRI* are both useful to localize the exact site of an aneurysm; assessment of renal artery involvement is essential to determine the type of operative approach.

• *Arteriography*: abdominal aneurysms may not necessarily show a widened lumen as the majority contain thrombus. Arteriography will demonstrate the distal circulation and relation of the renal arteries to the aneurysm.

TYPES OF ANEURYSM

• Traumatic.

• Congential: most commonly affects the intracranial circulation in the region of the circle of Willis ('berry aneurysm').

• Inflammatory: infection or abscess around the aorta leads to weakening of the wall.

• Dissecting: usually due to a tear in a weakened intimal wall in the thoracic aorta; predisposing factors include hypertension and Marfan's syndrome. Retrograde dissection can involve the coronary arteries, aortic valve and the pericardial sac. CT or MRI may detect an intimal flap separating the two lumina, MRI being the more sensitive investigation.

• Degenerative: commonest sites are the abdominal aorta, iliacs, femorals and popliteals.

• Poststenotic: distal to arterial narrowing, such as coarctation.

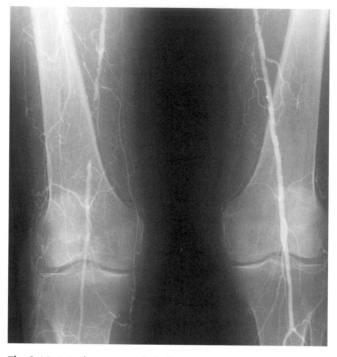

Fig. 3.14 Arteriogram: occluded segment in the right femoral artery.

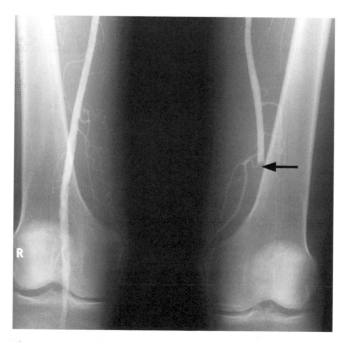

Fig. 3.15 Femoral embolus: sharp contrast cut off in the left femoral artery (arrow) due to embolus. Note the poor collateral circulation.

PERIPHERAL VASCULAR DISEASE

Arterial insufficiency commonly develops in the lower limbs from atheromatous involvement of the aorta and lower-limb arteries. Pain in the calves or buttocks on exercise (intermittent claudication), cold limbs and ulceration are the commonest clinical features. Predisposing causes include diabetes and smoking.

RADIOLOGICAL INVESTIGATIONS

Doppler ultrasound; arteriography; MRI.

RADIOLOGICAL FEATURES

Ultrasound will diagnose major occlusions but arteriography is required for the accurate visualization of diseased vessels, stenoses and occlusions; resolution of MR angiography has recently shown such significant improvements that it may eventually replace conventional arteriography.

TREATMENT

- Balloon angioplasty.
- Metallic stent insertion under radiological control.
- Surgical bypass grafts: aorto-iliac, femoropopliteal and femorofemoral.

ARTERIAL EMBOLUS

An arterial embolus occurs when blood clot, originating elsewhere in the cardiovascular system, travels more peripherally and occludes an artery. The lower limbs are affected in the majority of cases. Symptoms are of rapid onset and consist of a cold, pale, numb leg with absent pulses distal to the occlusion. Predisposing factors include recent myocardial infarction with mural thrombus and atrial fibrillation. If there is co-existing vascular disease, a diagnosis of acute thrombosis should be considered.

RADIOLOGICAL FEATURES

Peripheral arteriography demonstrates the contrast column in the artery with a sharp, well-defined cut-off point, usually a convex upper border projecting into the lumen of the vessel. Further evidence of an acute episode is provided by a deficient collateral circulation.

TREATMENT

- Surgical embolectomy.
- Thrombolysis: perfusion of streptokinase or tissue plasminogen activator (TPA) directly into the arterial thrombus in order to lyse the clot.

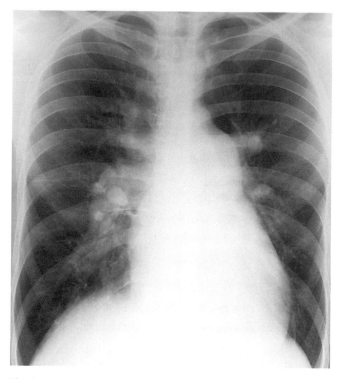

Fig. 3.16 Pulmonary hypertension: bilateral hilar vascular enlargement and prominence of the pulmonary outflow tract.

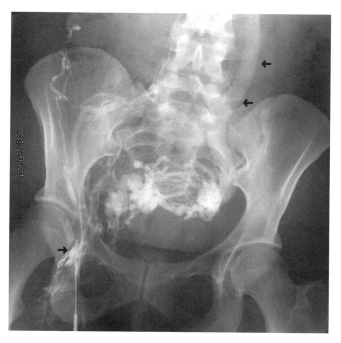

Fig. 3.17 Venogram with contrast injection in the right femoral vein (→) showing a complete occlusion of the inferior vena cava and a collateral circulation via a hypertrophied ascending lumbar vein (←).

PULMONARY ARTERIAL HYPERTENSION

Pulmonary arterial hypertension refers to increased pulmonary artery pressure from its normal value of 25/10 mmHg to greater than 30/15 mmHg.

RADIOLOGICAL FEATURES

Hypertension has to be quite marked before changes on a chest X-ray.
- Cardiac enlargement with right ventricular hypertrophy.
- Dilatation of the pulmonary hilar vessels with distal attenuation.
- Distension of the main pulmonary artery with a bulge below the aortic knuckle.

CAUSES

- Increased pulmonary blood flow in congenital heart disease.
- Obstruction of the pulmonary circulation, e.g. pulmonary emboli, parenchymal lung disease.
- Secondary to pulmonary venous hypertension from left-heart failure or mitral stenosis.

SUPERIOR AND INFERIOR VENA CAVA OBSTRUCTION

The superior (SVC) and inferior vena cava (IVC) may obstruct from many causes resulting in distal venous distension.

PRESENTATION

- SVC obstruction: facial and neck oedema, visible collateral veins.
- IVC obstruction: lower limb oedema, scrotal oedema.

RADIOLOGICAL INVESTIGATIONS

- *Doppler ultrasound*: verifies decreased or lack of a blood flow pattern.
- *CT/MRI*: confirms occlusion and often identifies the cause.
- *Venography*: demonstrates anatomical detail, especially useful if stenting is to be considered.

CAUSES OF SVC OBSTRUCTION

- Neoplastic: bronchial carcinoma, lymphoma, radiotherapy.
- Benign: mediastinal disease due to tuberculosis, sarcoid.

CAUSES OF IVC OBSTRUCTION

- Tumour invasion from abdominal neoplasms, most commonly renal.
- Retroperitoneal fibrosis; radiotherapy.

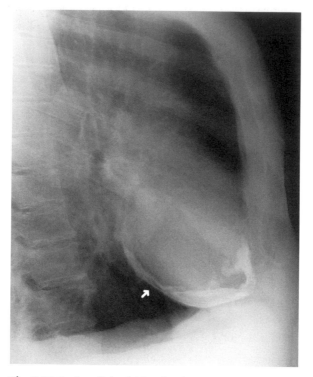

Fig. 3.18 Pericardial calcification (arrow).

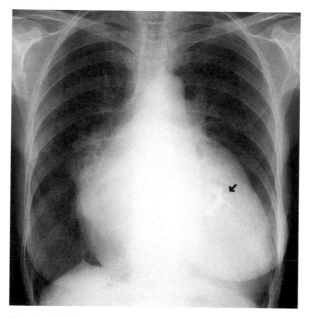

Fig. 3.19 Enlarged heart resulting from mitral valvular disease showing valve calcification (arrow).

CARDIAC CALCIFICATION

PERICARDIAL CALCIFICATION

Usually follows pericarditis: tuberculosis, rheumatoid arthritis, pyogenic, viral or rheumatic fever; the aetiology may be unknown.

MYOCARDIAL CALCIFICATION

Occurs typically at the apex of the left ventricle; the common causes are myocardial infarction and ventricular aneurysm.

VALVE CALCIFICATION

Calcification in the valves is common, but has to be quite extensive before being evident on plain films. Calcification usually means an element of stenosis, with the aortic and mitral valves most commonly affected. Causes include atheroma, rheumatic valvular disease and congenital bicuspid valve.

AORTIC-WALL CALCIFICATION

May be present in atheroma, in the wall of an aneurysm or represent syphilitic aortitis (ascending aorta).

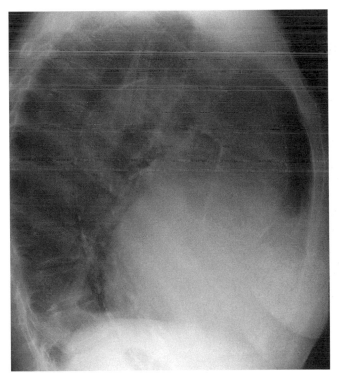

Fig. 3.20 Aortic-wall calcification.

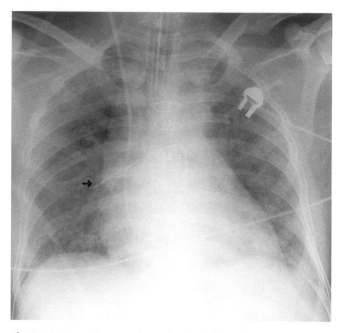

Fig. 3.21 Swan–Ganz catheter in the right pulmonary artery (arrow) and endotracheal tube in a patient after cardiac surgery (note ECG leads).

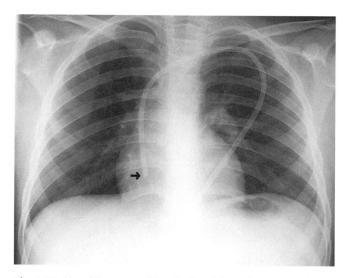

Fig. 3.22 Tip of the central line in the right atrium (arrow).

TUBE AND CATHETER PLACEMENT

ENDOTRACHEAL TUBE

The tip should be positioned 5–7 cm above the carina. When sited too far, the endotracheal tube may advance into a main bronchus, causing collapse of the opposite lung.

CENTRAL LINE

Inserted via the jugular or subclavian veins into a large intrathoracic vein. For accurate measurement of right atrial pressure, the tip of the catheter must lie in a large intrathoracic vein such as the superior vena cava.

SWAN–GANZ CATHETER

The catheter is inserted via the jugular, subclavian or femoral vein and manipulated through the right heart into either the right or left pulmonary artery. The end-diastolic left-ventricular pressure is estimated from a reading taken at the distal tip of the catheter.

NASOGASTRIC TUBE

The radio-opaque tip should be visualized in the region of the stomach on plain films. An X-ray is usually necessary to ensure that the tube is not mal-positioned, especially into the trachea or bronchus.

PACING WIRE

Pacemaker leads are placed through the subclavian or internal jugular veins into the right side of the heart, with the tip implanted at the apex of the right ventricle, whereas dual-lead pacemakers have their ends positioned in the right atrium and ventricle.

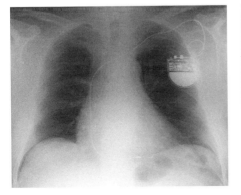

Fig. 3.23 Single-pacing lead.

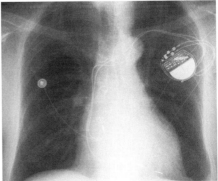

Fig. 3.24 Dual-pacing leads.

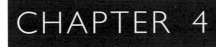
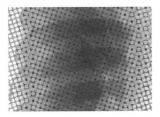

CHAPTER 4

Gastrointestinal Tract

GASTROINTESTINAL TRACT INVESTIGATIONS

- *Plain films.* Plain films may be helpful in detecting intestinal obstruction, extraluminal free gas and abdominal calcification.
- *Barium swallow.* The main indications are dysphagia and symptoms of gastro-oesophageal reflux. The oesophagus is visualized under fluoroscopy as the patient swallows barium and studied for incoordinate peristalsis, motility problems or structural abnormalities. Water-soluble contrast agents are used in suspected oesophageal rupture.
- *Barium meal.* The patient is fasted overnight for the examination. Double contrast is obtained by introduction of gas into the stomach using effervescent powders. Glucagon or Buscopan administered intravenously suppresses motility and improves film quality. The examination is controlled under fluoroscopy, spot films being obtained in different projections of the gas and barium-filled stomach. The gastro-oesophageal junction is observed for reflux.
- *Barium follow-through.* Transit of barium is observed through the small bowel after 200–300 ml of barium is swallowed. Full-length abdominal films are taken every half hour until barium reaches the terminal ileum and large bowel.
- *Small-bowel enema.* This is a specific study of the small bowel, with visualization superior to a follow-through examination. A specially designed tube is passed nasally and manoeuvred into the duodenojejunal flexure under fluoroscopic control. Subsequently, approximately I litre of dilute barium is infused through this tube until a continuous column of barium reaches the terminal ileum. The technique is more rapid and exact in the detection of small-bowel pathology than a barium follow-through examination, although more unpleasant for the patient.

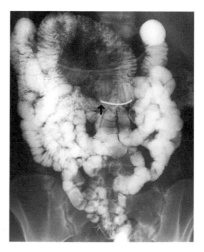

Fig. 4.1 Normal small-bowel enema. Note the tip of the tube in the jejunum (arrow).

Barium enema. The principal indications for this study of the large bowel are for a change in bowel habit, haemorrhage, investigation of an abdominal mass or location of the site of large-bowel obstruction. Contraindications to this procedure are toxic megacolon, pseudomembranous colitis, recent radiotherapy or full-thickness bowel-wall biopsy. A clean colon is essential and laxatives are administered the day before the examination. Barium is run into the colon by means of a tube placed in the rectum and spot films obtained under fluoroscopic control. Air introduced into the large bowel produces a double-contrast examination. A rare, recognized complication is bowel perforation, which may result in peritonitis.

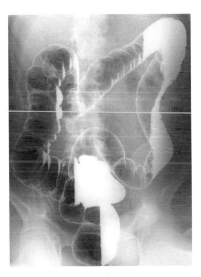

Fig. 4.2 Normal barium enema with barium (white) and air contrast (black).

Isotope scanning. Technetium-99 m pertechnetate may be used for studies of gastric emptying, gastrointestinal haemorrhage and also in the detection of a Meckel's diverticulum (accumulation in ectopic gastric mucosa).

Arteriography. Contrast injection into the superior and inferior mesenteric arteries may pinpoint the source of acute small- or large-bowel haemorrhage. Bleeding has to be fairly brisk, however, at 1–2 ml/min.

Computed tomography (CT) scanning. Uses in the gastrointestinal tract include:
- staging of tumours for secondary deposits and adjacent infiltration;
- localizing abscesses;
- as an aid to biopsy and drainage procedures.

PLAIN ABDOMEN FILM

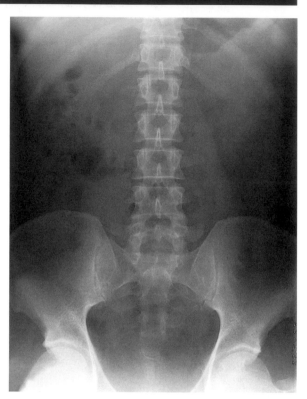

Fig. 4.3 Normal plain abdomen.

The routine projection used is the supine one. Erect abdomen films may illustrate air/fluid levels in obstruction, and free gas under the diaphragm in perforation although, in the latter, an erect chest film is more appropriate.

When assessing an abdominal film, a study of three principal aspects will encompass the majority of abnormal findings: bowel gas pattern; areas of calcification; skeletal abnormalities.

BOWEL GAS PATTERN

A marked variation exists in the amount of bowel gas in normal individuals, usually some gas being noted in the stomach, small and large bowel. Bowel gas pattern should be evaluated with particular reference to dilatation. Generally, the small bowel lies in a central position characterized by folds or valvulae conniventes forming complete bands across the bowel. The large bowel, however, is situated peripherally, the haustral pattern forming incomplete transverse bands. Small-bowel dilatation is considered to be present if the width exceeds 3 cm. Conditions that may be diagnosed by an alteration in the bowel gas pattern are: small-bowel obstruction; large-bowel obstruction; paralytic ileus; caecal volvulus; sigmoid volvulus; toxic megacolon. Gas may be noted outside the bowel lumen in the biliary system, urinary tract, subphrenic abscess, colon wall or abdominal abscess, but this is often difficult to interpret.

Calcification

A great majority of calcifications are of no real clinical significance: costal cartilage, pelvic vein phleboliths, mesenteric lymph nodes and vascular calcification. Some abnormal areas are shown in the figure below.

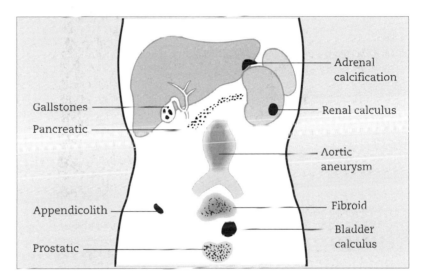

Fig. 4.4 Pathological calcifications in the abdomen.

Skeletal abnormalities

Skeletal abnormalities that may be shown on plain abdominal films are degenerative changes in the spine or hips; bony metastases; Paget's disease; sacroilitis; vertebral body collapse.

Other abnormalities

Hepatosplenomegaly; mass lesions seen by distortion of the bowel gas pattern; soft-tissue masses arising from intra-abdominal and pelvic organs.

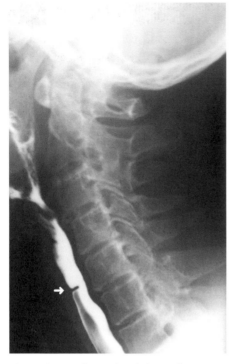

Fig. 4.5 Oesophageal web (arrow).

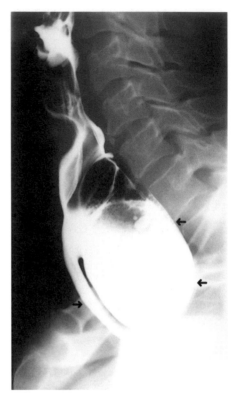

Fig. 4.6 Large pharyngeal pouch (←) containing stagnant food residue. The upper oesophagus (→)is pushed forwards by the pouch.

OESOPHAGEAL WEB

An oesophageal web is a thin membranous band arising from the anterior upper oesophageal wall, especially from the pharyngo-oesophageal junction. It is covered with normal-appearing mucosa and protrudes posteriorly to a varying extent. Webs may be multiple and there is a recognized association with postcricoid carcinoma.

PRESENTATION

Dysphagia; incidental finding; iron-deficiency anaemia (Plummer–Vinson syndrome).

RADIOLOGICAL FEATURES

A barium study reveals an anterior fine linear filling defect on the barium filled upper oesophagus. Webs are best seen on the lateral projection.

TREATMENT

Oesophagoscopy usually ruptures the web and also excludes other oesophageal pathology.

PHARYNGEAL POUCH

A pharyngeal pouch results from a posterior mucosal protrusion arising from between the vertical and horizontal fibres of the inferior constrictor of the pharynx, just above the cricopharyngeus. Lateral pouches or diverticula are rare. Diverticula may be found in any part of the oesophagus; aspiration pneumonia is a recognized complication.

PRESENTATION

Dysphagia; repeated attacks of aspiration pneumonia; food regurgitation; halitosis; palpable neck mass.

RADIOLOGICAL FEATURES

Plain films of the cervical region in the erect position may show a fluid level in the pouch. A barium swallow reveals the pouch filling posteriorly from the oesophageal wall, connected by a relatively narrow neck and often containing stagnating food residue.

TREATMENT

Surgical resection, using an external approach or by endoscopic technique.

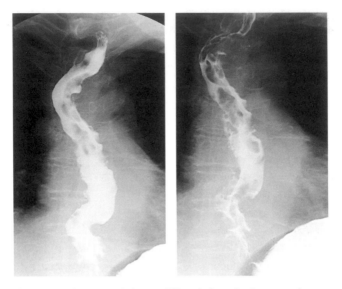

Fig. 4.7 Varices: serpiginous filling defects in the oesophagus.

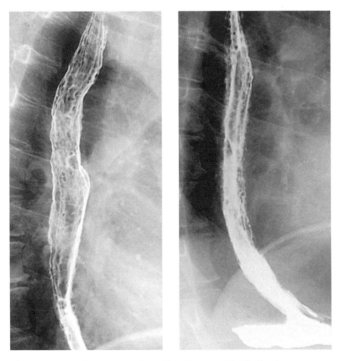

Fig. 4.8 Irregular mucosal outline in monilial infection.

OESOPHAGEAL VARICES

Oesophageal varices are venous anastomotic collateral veins, usually resulting from portal venous hypertension or portal-vein obstruction. They commonly develop as a result of liver cirrhosis, are confined to the lower two-thirds of the oesophagus and are often associated with gastric varices ('uphill varices' with portosystemic shunting: collateral blood flow via the azygos vein into the superior vena cava (SVC) from the portal vein). Varices in the upper oesophagus can develop from superior vena cava obstruction ('downhill varices': collaterals from SVC, via azygos vein into inferior vena cava (IVC) or the portal vein).

RADIOLOGICAL FEATURES

Endoscopy is the investigation of choice but a barium swallow can delineate the large submucosal veins in the oesophagus and gastric fundus in many cases. On the barium-filled column, varices are seen as serpiginous tortuous filling defects. Spiral CT scanning with contrast may also identify the varices.

MONILIASIS

Fungal infection of the oesophagus with *Candida* occurs in patients who are debilitated, immunosuppressed or on broad-spectrum antibiotic therapy. The incidence of pharyngeal and oesophageal candidiasis is particularly high in patients with acquired immune deficiency syndrome (AIDS).

PRESENTATION

Painful dysphagia; chest pain.

RADIOLOGICAL FEATURES

On barium-swallow examination, the margins of the oesophagus are irregular with small mucosal plaques, seen as filling defects. The mucosa may be ulcerated with a cobblestone appearance.

DIFFERENTIAL OF AN IRREGULAR OESOPHAGUS

- Oesophagitis following caustic ingestion: in the acute stage, atonic, ulcerated oesophagus with subsequent stricture formation.
- Reflux oesophagitis.
- Herpetic oesophagitis.

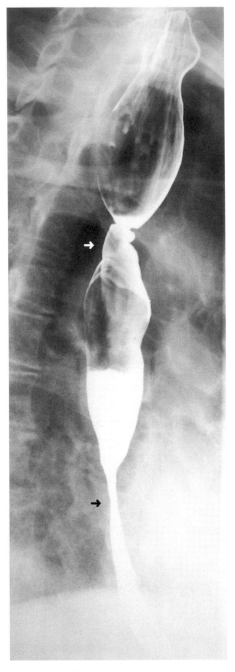

Fig. 4.10 Achalasia: dilated tortuous oesophagus with narrowing at the gastro-oesophageal junction (arrow).

Fig. 4.9 Multiple benign strictures (arrows) from caustic soda ingestion; the mucosal outline appears smooth.

BENIGN OESOPHAGEAL STRICTURE

Benign oesophageal strictures have numerous aetiologies, and often present with dysphagia. Carcinoma should always be suspected in the presence of an oesophageal stricture, as radiological appearances can sometimes be misleading.

RADIOLOGICAL FEATURES

These depend on the cause. In the acute stage, there may be oedema and ulceration of the oesophagus. Chronic benign strictures have smooth tapering margins, often with proximal dilatation.

CAUSES

The usual cause is peptic stricture secondary to reflux; others include: corrosive stricture: tend to be long and smooth in the chronic phase; achalasia: found at the level of the diaphragm; skin disorders: epidermolysis bullosa and pemphigus; traumatic: from prolonged indwelling nasogastric tube, radiotherapy; scleroderma.

ACHALASIA

A functional disorder of motility in achalasia causes an inability of the lower oesophageal sphincter to relax. Dysphagia, weight loss and regurgitation of stagnating oesophageal contents are the commonest presenting symptoms. Complications include recurrent pulmonary aspiration and an increased incidence of oesophageal carcinoma.

RADIOLOGICAL FEATURES

• *Chest film*: the dilated oesophagus may be rendered visible by retained food contents giving rise to a widened mediastinum. Reduced air in the stomach produces a small or absent gastric air bubble. Aspiration into the lungs may lead to chronic basal changes.

• *Barium swallow*: shows gross oesophageal dilatation and tortuosity, usually with retained food residue. There is poor peristaltic activity, with narrowing at the oesophagogastric junction due to failure of relaxation of the lower sphincter.

TREATMENT

• Balloon dilatation in the narrowed segment to rupture the muscle fibres.
• Oesophagomyotomy (Heller's operation).

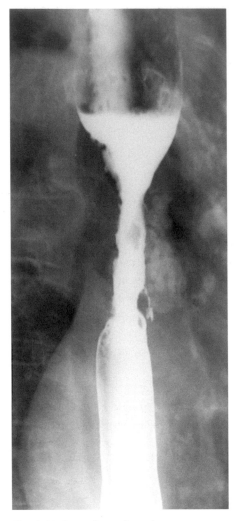

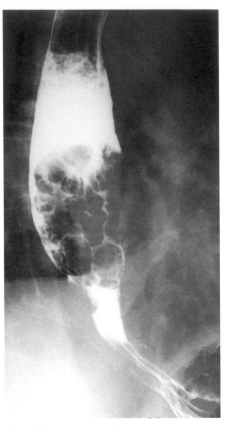

Fig. 4.12 Oesophageal carcinoma: polypoidal type with an intraluminal mass.

Fig. 4.11 Oesophageal carcinoma: irregular narrowing with mucosal destruction.

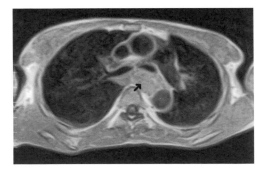

Fig. 4.13 MRI of the chest shows the extent of an oesophageal carcinoma (arrow).

OESOPHAGEAL CARCINOMA

Carcinoma of the oesophagus, usually a squamous cell type, occurs most frequently in the distal third of the oesophagus and is much more common in males. Predisposing factors include achalasia, Barrett's oesophagus (columnar epithelium lining the oesophagus), caustic stricture and the Plummer–Vinson syndrome.

PRESENTATION

- Progressive dysphagia, often painful.
- Weight loss.

RADIOLOGICAL INVESTIGATIONS

- *Barium swallow*: the initial investigation of choice.
- *CT scanning thorax*: assesses tumour confinement to the wall or extraluminal spread into the adjacent mediastinum and secondary spread to supraclavicular nodes.
- *CT scanning abdomen or ultrasound abdomen*: to search for secondary deposits in the liver and para-aortic nodes.

RADIOLOGICAL FEATURES

On barium examiation:
- Polypoidal type: an intraluminal mass protrudes out into the oesophageal lumen causing a filling defect in the barium column.
- Infiltrative type: the tumour spreads under the oesophageal mucosa without extending into the lumen, causing narrowing. Later there is mucosal infiltration resulting in ulceration and an irregular outline to the oesophagus.

Occasionally, there is a tracheo- or broncho-oesophageal fistula.

TREATMENT

Prognosis is dismal with <10% 5-year survival regardless of treatment. At the time of presentation, most have mediastinal or distant spread; therapy is usually palliative.
- Surgical resection: when there is no mediastinal or distant spread. A postoperative check of the integrity of the anastomosis can be made with a water-soluble contrast swallow examination.
- Palliative radiotherapy: squamous cell carcinomas are responsive with rapid relief of symptoms.
- Palliative intubation: either through an endoscope or metallic stent insertion under fluoroscopic control.

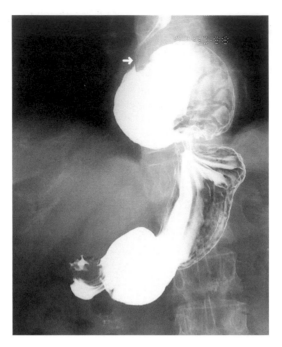

Fig. 4.14 Sliding hiatus hernia: the gastro-oesophageal junction (arrow) is above the diaphragm.

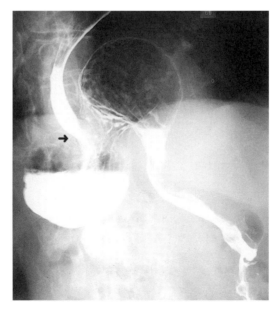

Fig. 4.15 Rolling hiatus hernia: the gastro-oesophageal junction (arrow) is in its normal position below the diaphragm.

HIATUS HERNIA

A hiatus hernia develops from protrusion of a portion of the stomach, through the oesophageal hiatus of the diaphragm, into the thorax. A broad spectrum of appearances arise, ranging from the whole stomach lying in the intrathoracic position to small herniations which slide back easily.

Sliding hiatus hernia. Most common type where the gastro-oesophageal junction and the stomach slide to lie above the diaphragm. There may be associated gastro-oesophageal reflux. Its incidence increases with age, and the hernia is usually reducible in the erect position.

Para-oesophageal hernia. Uncommon and usually irreducible. The gastro-oesophageal junction lies in a normal position with the stomach herniating alongside the oesophagus. There is no associated reflux.

PRESENTATION

- Heartburn: worse on lying flat.
- Dysphagia: due either to inflammatory change or stricture.
- Retrosternal pain: can be mistaken for cardiac pain.
- Anaemia.

RADIOLOGICAL FEATURES

- *Chest X-ray*: may demonstrate a soft-tissue mass in the posterior mediastinum, behind the cardiac shadow. An air/fluid level is sometimes noted in the hernia.
- *Barium swallow*: readily shows the herniation. The patient needs to be examined in the 'head-down' position to demonstrate small herniations with or without gastro-oesophageal reflux.

COMPLICATIONS

- Oesophagitis: inflammatory changes secondary to acid regurgitation.
- Oesophageal ulceration: associated with reflux.
- Oesophageal stricture: healing by fibrosis can lead to stricture formation. When this complication arises, an endoscopy is needed to exclude a stricture secondary to carcinoma.
- Anaemia.
- Incarceration, though rare, may lead to obstruction, perforation, strangulation, haemorrhage or respiratory symptoms.

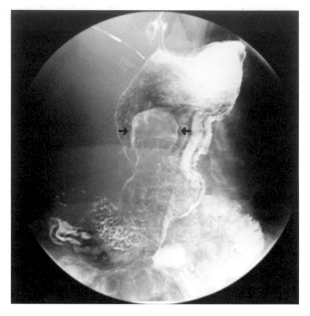

Fig. 4.16 Leiomyoma: well-defined benign tumour (arrows).

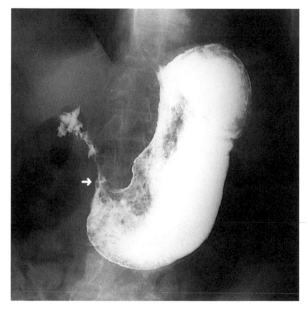

Fig. 4.17 Gastric outlet obstruction due to carcinoma of the pyloric antral region (arrow).

LEIOMYOMA

A leiomyoma is a benign tumour arising from the muscle layers of the intestinal tract. It is the most frequent benign tumour of the stomach after a gastric polyp.

RADIOLOGICAL FEATURES

On barium examination there is a smooth well-defined mass, with overlying stretched mucosa, projecting into the stomach. These benign neoplasms often ulcerate with a central ulcer crater.

COMPLICATIONS

Gastrointestinal bleeding; malignant change to leiomyosarcoma.

DIFFERENTIAL DIAGNOSIS

This is from other benign tumours arising from the gastric wall: lipoma; schwannoma from nerve sheaths; fibroma.

GASTRIC OUTLET OBSTRUCTION

Vomiting, weight loss and electrolyte imbalance due to loss of gastric acid are the main clinical features when the outlet of the stomach is obstructed.

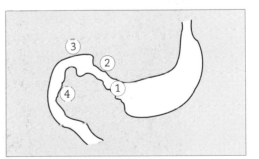

Fig. 4.18 Causes of gastric outlet obstruction. 1, Gastric antrum: ulcer or carcinoma; 2, pyloric canal: adult hypertrophic stenosis (rare); 3, duodenal cap: ulceration with scarring of the duodenal cap; 4, duodenal loop: pancreatic carcinoma or duodenal carcinoma.

RADIOLOGICAL FEATURES

The stomach is distended and often enlarged with an increased amount of resting gastric juice. A barium meal demonstrates food residue in the stomach, with a delay in barium leaving the stomach or duodenum, depending on the level and degree of obstruction. Peristaltic activity may be increased, but is more commonly diminished and the stomach is atonic. Narrowing and irregularity occur from fibrotic change, spasm and oedema or due to malignant infiltration.

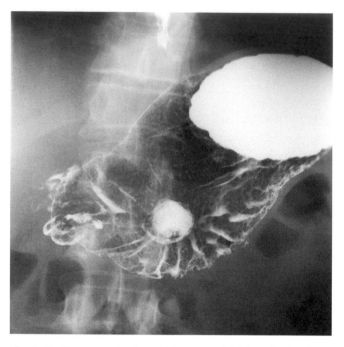

Fig. 4.19 Giant gastric ulcer with mucosal folds radiating into the ulcer.

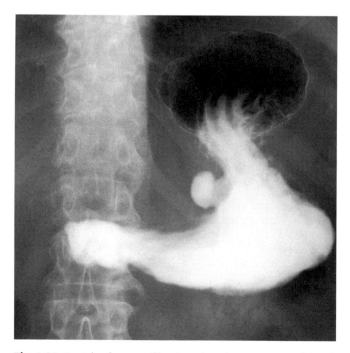

Fig. 4.20 Gastric ulcer: profile view showing an outpouching from the lesser curve.

GASTRIC ULCER

Gastric ulcers occur most commonly on the lesser curve, but may arise in any part of the stomach. Endoscopy is the preferred technique although a barium study is also accurate. Predisposing causes include smoking, psychological stress, non-steroidal analgesics and steroids. Multiple gastric ulcers are found in the Zollinger–Ellison syndrome.

PRESENTATION

Nausea; anorexia; vomiting; weight loss; upper abdominal pain; complications such as perforation, haematemesis or melaena.

RADIOLOGICAL FEATURES

On barium examination, *en face* views may show a pool of barium collecting in the ulcer crater on the dependent wall, with mucosal folds radiating directly to the ulcer. On profile views, the ulcer appears as an outpouching from the gastric wall.

• Benign ulcer: smooth radiating folds, and projection of the ulcer out of the gastric wall.

• Malignant ulcer: a shallow ulcer, irregular in contour, which does not protrude beyond the confines of the stomach. There may be an associated mass with destruction of the mucosal pattern.

COMPLICATIONS

See 'Duodenal ulcer' (p. 105).

TREATMENT

• Medical: the majority of gastric ulcers are benign, and if obviously so, can be treated medically with serial follow-up to complete healing. If there is any doubt, then endoscopy with biopsy is suggested.

• Surgical: partial gastrectomy.

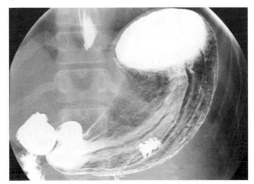

Fig. 4.21 Normal stomach with barium and air contrast.

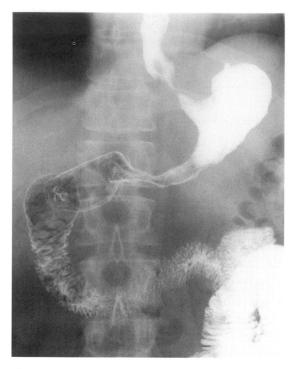

Fig. 4.22 Gastric carcinoma: linitis plastica type with a contracted stomach.

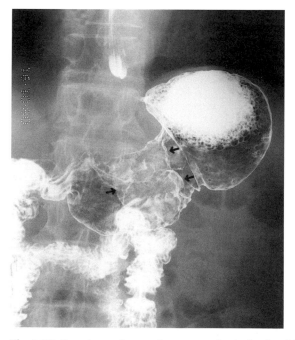

Fig. 4.23 Gastric carcinoma: large mass in the body of the stomach (arrows).

GASTRIC CARCINOMA

There has been a general decrease in the incidence of gastric carcinoma, although there remains a very high prevalence of the disease in the Japanese population. Predisposing factors include pernicious anaemia, chronic atrophic gastritis, adenomatous polyps and previous partial gastrectomy. An association with *Helicobacter pylori* infection is being explored.

PRESENTATION

Dyspepsia; anorexia; nausea and vomiting; weight loss; haematemesis or melaena.

RADIOLOGICAL INVESTIGATIONS

- Endoscopy or barium meal.
- Ultrasound and CT for pre-operative evaluation.

RADIOLOGICAL FEATURES

Barium meal examination may reveal the following forms of gastric carcinoma.
- Polypoidal type: soft-tissue mass causing a filling defect in the stomach.
- Ulcerating type: the ulcerating area is confined to within the margin of the stomach.
- Diffuse infiltrating type: diffuse submucosal infiltration with muscle invasion leads to a small rigid stomach with poor distensibility: linitis plastica or 'leather bottle stomach'.
- Local infiltrating type: a focal area of mucosal irregularity and narrowing at the site of the tumour.

TREATMENT

At the time of diagnosis, gastric carcinoma is usually advanced, hence an extremely poor 5-year survival rate: total gastrectomy as a possible curative procedure; palliative partial gastrectomy for obstruction.

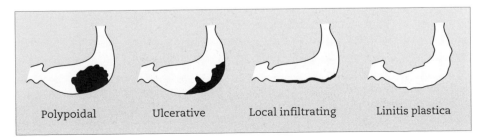

| Polypoidal | Ulcerative | Local infiltrating | Linitis plastica |

Fig. 4.24 Types of gastric carcinoma.

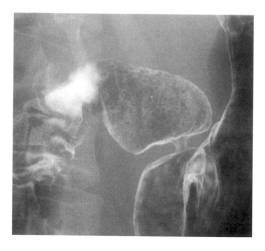

Fig. 4.25 Normal duodenal bulb (air-filled).

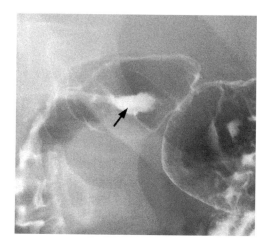

Fig. 4.26 Duodenal ulcer crater filling with barium (arrow).

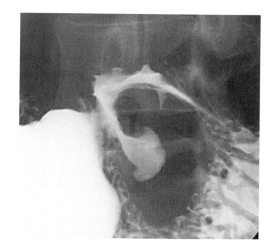

Fig. 4.27 Scarred and deformed duodenal bulb due to chronic ulceration (barium-filled).

DUODENAL ULCER

Duodenal ulcers occur more commonly than gastric ulcers. The most frequent site for a duodenal ulcer is in the proximal duodenum, called the 'cap' or 'bulb'. Postbulbar ulcers are rare.

RADIOLOGICAL FEATURES

Endoscopy is the investigation of choice, though a barium meal examination is still frequently performed. Diagnosis of a duodenal ulcer depends on the demonstration of a crater or niche, into which the barium pools. The ulcer crater can occur on either the anterior or posterior wall of the duodenum and occasionally ulceration may develop in the postbulbar area. Chronic ulceration leads to fibrosis, scarring, narrowing and deformity of the duodenum. Duodenitis and mucosal ulcerations may prove difficult to demonstrate on a barium study.

COMPLICATIONS

• Perforation. An ulcer may erode through the wall with perforation and escape of intraluminal contents into the abdominal cavity. This may result in free air in the peritoneal cavity, shown on plain abdominal and erect chest films by a crescent of gas under the diaphragm.

• Haemorrhage. Erosion of the ulcer into a vessel may lead to significant haemorrhage, with either haematemesis or melaena. Endoscopy is helpful to pinpoint the source. Angiography may be used, if endoscopy is not satisfactory, to localize the source in active bleeding.

• Gastric outlet obstruction. Due to fibrosis, scarring and narrowing.

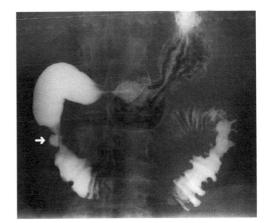

Fig. 4.28 Postbulbar ulcer (arrow).

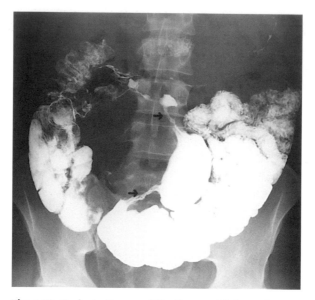

Fig. 4.29 Crohn's disease of the ileum with irregular narrowed segments (arrows).

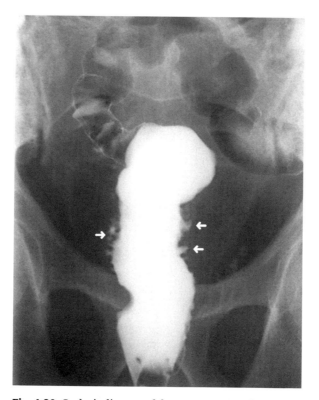

Fig. 4.30 Crohn's disease of the rectum: note the deep ulceration (arrows).

CROHN'S DISEASE

Crohn's disease, a chronic inflammatory condition of unknown aetiology, can affect any part of the alimentary tract from the oesophagus to rectum, but most commonly involves the terminal ileum and small bowel.

RADIOLOGICAL FEATURES

The terminal ileum is the site most commonly affected in the small bowel, although the large bowel is also frequently affected and may be solely involved. On a barium study, the following may be seen in the small bowel.
- Deep ulceration (rose thorn) affecting the entire bowel wall.
- Cobblestone appearance to the mucosa, caused by ulcers separated by raised areas of oedema.
- Loss of peristalsis, thickening and rigidity of bowel wall; separation of small bowel loops due to the thickness of their walls.
- Stricture formation from oedema and fibrosis (string sign of Kantor).

In colonic Crohn's disease the most frequent features found are deep ulceration, apthous ulcers and discontinuous involvement with normal intervening bowel (skip lesions).

COMPLICATIONS

- Subacute obstruction as a result of stricture formation.
- Abscess formation, sometimes leading to bowel perforation.
- Malabsorption from extensive small-bowel involvement and interruption of the enterohepatic circulation.
- Perianal inflammatory changes may result from abscess or fissure.
- Fistulae to large bowel, vagina, bladder, perineum and abdominal wall from inflamed small bowel adhering to adjacent structures.

Extrahepatic

Gallstones; sclerosing cholangitis; arthritis; oxalate and uric acid urinary calculi; uveitis.

DIFFERENTIAL OF SMALL BOWEL NARROWING

Adhesions; Crohn's disease; carcinoma (the duodenum is the most frequent site in the small bowel); metastases; radiotherapy; ischaemia; tuberculosis.

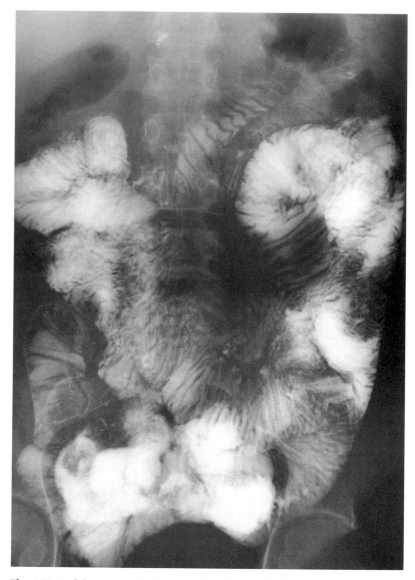

Fig. 4.31 Malabsorption: dilatation of small bowel with thickening of mucosal folds.

MALABSORPTION

Malabsorption is characterized by a deficient intestinal absorption of essential nutrients.

RADIOLOGICAL FEATURES

Radiological examination of the small bowel is by a barium follow-through examination or a small-bowel enema. Although radiological investigation may reveal specific causes, such as Crohn's disease, fistulae or diverticula, the prime importance of radiology is to identify a malabsorption pattern. This is usually not specific for a diagnosis, and a jejunal biopsy will be required.

The following features may be shown on a barium examination:

- dilatation of small bowel;
- prominence of small-bowel transverse bands, the valvulae conniventes;
- thickening of bowel wall, with separation of adjacent loops.

CAUSES

There are a large number of causes, some of which are:

Intraluminal:

- pancreatic insufficiency: pancreatitis, carcinoma and cystic fibrosis;
- biliary insufficiency: liver disease or biliary obstruction.

Mucosal: extensive damage or infiltration of mucosal surface: coeliac disease (commonest cause), Crohn's disease and radiation enteritis.

Anatomical: fistulae, gastrectomy, small-bowel resection or small-bowel diverticulosis.

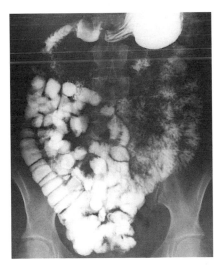

Fig. 4.32 Normal barium follow-through examination of the small bowel. Barium has passed into the ascending colon.

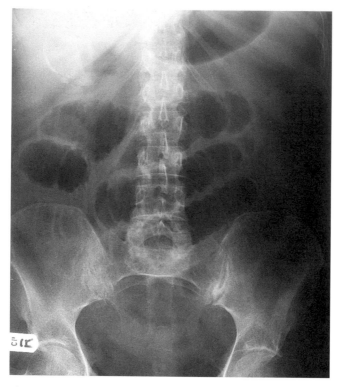

Fig. 4.33 Small bowel obstruction: distended small bowel and absence of gas shadows in the colon.

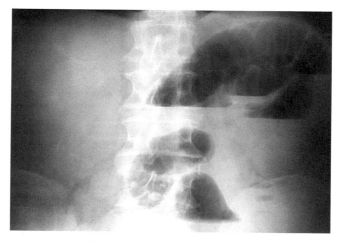

Fig. 4.34 Erect film demonstrating multiple small bowel air/fluid levels.

SMALL-BOWEL OBSTRUCTION

Mechanical small-bowel obstruction develops when there is impairment to the onward flow of bowel contents.

RADIOLOGICAL FEATURES

Gas and fluid accumulating proximal to the site of obstruction cause progressive dilatation of small bowel. Some features on plain abdominal films are:

• Central distended loops of small bowel, often >3 cm in diameter.

• Transverse stripes of the valvulae conniventes generally extend across the whole of the small bowel; in the large bowel, the haustrae do not cross the diameter of the colon.

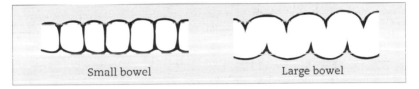

Small bowel   Large bowel

Fig. 4.35 Appearance of valvulae conniventes in the small bowel and haustral pattern in the large bowel.

• Absence of gas in the large bowel. If gas is still present, it indicates that obstruction is recent or that it is incomplete.

• When obstruction is high, such as the duodenum or upper jejunum, the above signs may be absent with lack of small-bowel distension or fluid levels.

• The site of obstruction can be predicted. If only a few dilated loops are found, then the obstruction is likely to be upper jejunum, but a large number of small-bowel loops indicates that obstruction is in the ileum: the greater the number of distended loops, the more distal the site of obstruction.

When plain abdominal films are equivocal, barium follow-through examination may identify the level of obstruction, the principal feature being a change in the calibre from the dilated segment to a collapsed distal small bowel. Barium should only be used if a colonic cause of obstruction has been excluded, as inspissated barium can turn an incomplete into a complete large-bowel obstruction. A barium enema is always 'safe' in any suspected obstruction.

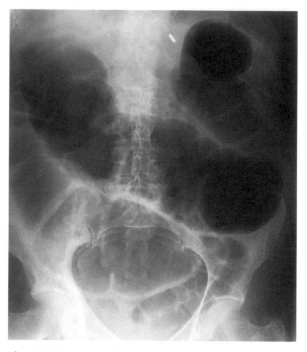

Fig. 4.36 Large bowel obstruction with a distended colon up to the splenic flexure.

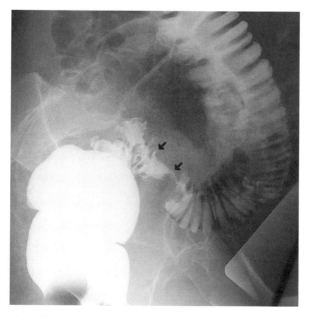

Fig. 4.37 Barium enema demonstrating a sigmoid carcinoma (arrows) as the cause of a large bowel obstruction.

LARGE-BOWEL OBSTRUCTION

Obstruction of the large bowel usually results from either a colonic carcinoma (often rectosigmoid) or diverticular disease.

RADIOLOGICAL FEATURES

Plain abdominal films are useful for the diagnosis of large-bowel obstruction. The basic principle of diagnosing gut obstruction is to detect bowel dilatation to a level beyond which there is collapse of bowel. The location of this transition point is not always easy to identify. The large bowel distends with its peripheral distribution and distinctive haustration. Fluid levels present in an erect position tend to be long, as compared to short levels in small-bowel obstruction. Features found on plain abdominal films vary depending on the state of the ileocaecal valve.

• *With closed ileocaecal valve.* Gas distension is limited to the large bowel with progressive dilatation, especially of the caecum. A risk of caecal perforation is present, particularly if the diameter is >9 cm.

• *With open ileocaecal valve.* Both large and small bowel distend, the appearances resembling a paralytic ileus.

In equivocal cases, a barium or water-soluble contrast enema can be performed prior to surgery: this locates the site of large-bowel obstruction and excludes a pseudo-obstruction.

CAUSES

• *Luminal*: faecal impaction.
• *Bowel wall*:
   neoplastic: carcinoma;
   inflammatory: Crohn's disease, ulcerative colitis, diverticular disease;
   infection: tuberculosis.
• *Extrinsic*:
   malignant mass, bladder or pelvic malignancy;
   volvulus;
   hernia.

Pseudo-obstruction. May be associated with conditions such as pneumonia, infarction and myxoedema. Plain films reveal progressive dilatation of the colon, the appearances resembling mechanical obstruction and a barium enema may be required to exclude this.

Paralytic ileus. Very common in the postoperative period due to cessation of intestinal peristaltic activity. Accumulation of gas and fluid contents result in dilatation of both small and large bowel.

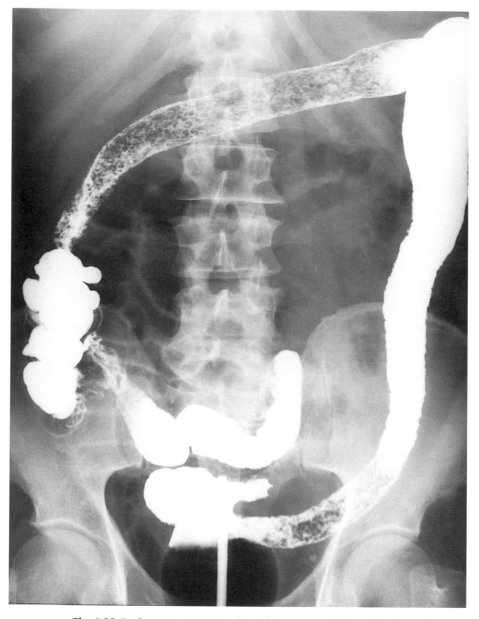

Fig. 4.38 Barium enema: extensive diffuse mucosal ulceration in the large bowel, with loss of the normal haustral pattern in ulcerative colitis.

ULCERATIVE COLITIS

Ulcerative colitis, an inflammatory disease of the large bowel, is characterized by diffuse mucosal damage with ulceration. The inflammatory reaction is limited to the mucosa and submucosa. An autoimmune state is a likely causative factor but the aetiology of the disease remains unknown.

RADIOLOGICAL INVESTIGATIONS

A plain abdominal film may occasionally show an abnormal segment of large bowel, especially when the complication of toxic megacolon arises. Colonoscopy is more accurate for assessment of the disease, but evaluation by barium enema is still widely practised.

RADIOLOGICAL FEATURES

The affected colon, almost always involving the rectum and sigmoid, shows blurring of the normally sharp outline. The mucosa appears granular with shallow ulceration in continuity from the rectum to a variable distance into the proximal colon, and may involve the whole colon (pancolitis). Associated loss of haustral pattern with fibrotic changes may give the bowel a tube-like appearance, the so-called 'lead pipe' or 'hose pipe' colon.

COMPLICATIONS

Colonic:
- Toxic megacolon: a plain abdominal film may demonstrate pronounced bowel distension with an irregular outline, especially of the transverse colon. Barium enema is contraindicated when this complication develops.
- Bowel perforation: in either severe disease or secondary to toxic megacolon.
- Haemorrhage: often profuse.
- Carcinoma: increased incidence especially when there is a pancolitis and the disease has been present for over 10 years.
- Stricture formation: may be multiple with a smooth outline.

Extracolonic:
- Sacroilitis; arthritis; uveitis; sclerosing cholangitis.

TREATMENT

- Medical: steroids, systemic and local application in large bowel; sulphasalazine and related drugs.
- Surgical: total proctocolectomy with ileo-anal anastomosis in severe disease with intractable symptoms.

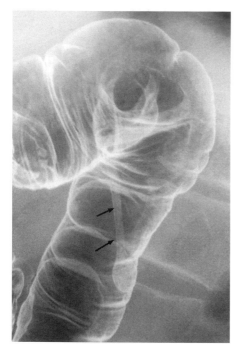

Fig. 4.39 Pedunculated colonic polyp.

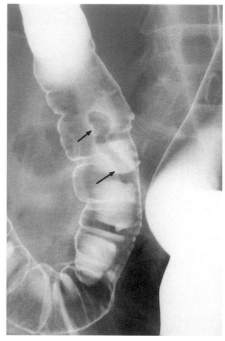

Fig. 4.40 Pedunculated polyp outlined by barium.

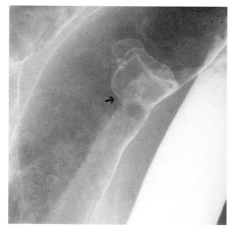

Fig. 4.41 Sessile polyp with a broad base.

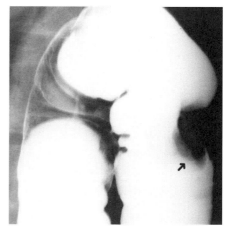

Fig. 4.42 Sessile polyp on a barium filled projection.

COLONIC POLYPS

Colonic polyps are localized mass lesions arising from the mucosa of the colon and protrude into the lumen. They may be broad based (sessile) or on a stalk (pedunculated) and occur anywhere in the colon. The majority of polyps are benign adenomas, especially those with long thin stalks.

RADIOLOGICAL FEATURES

Meticulous bowel preparation is needed as residual faeces and mucus greatly interfere with the correct diagnosis of colonic lesions. Double-contrast barium enema examination may demonstrate the polyp as a filling defect on the barium-filled views, or the polyp may be outlined by barium on the air-filled projections.

COMPLICATIONS

Malignancy in a polyp should be considered if there is:
- irregularity at the base or periphery;
- a flat lesion with a broader base than height;
- growth on serial examinations;
- a polyp > 10 mm.

TREATMENT

Small polyps can be snared and removed at colonoscopy; perforation and haemorrhage are infrequent complications of this procedure; larger lesions need formal surgical resection.

ADDITIONAL FEATURES

Multiple polyps may be found in the following.
- Familial adenomatous polyposis: an autosomal dominant inherited disease with multiple polyps, which become clinically apparent in the second decade. The risk of malignancy developing is almost 100%.
- Peutz–Jeghers syndrome: polyps are hamartomas with no malignant potential.
- Inflammatory bowel disease: in ulcerative colitis, less commonly Crohn's disease, areas of mucosal hyperplasia may be present (pseudopolyps).

CLASSIFICATION

- Neoplastic: adenoma, adenocarcinoma.
- Hamartomatous: Peutz–Jeghers syndrome.
- Inflammatory: Crohn's disease, ulcerative colitis. Hyperplastic over-growth of regenerating mucosa produces inflammatory pseudopolyps.

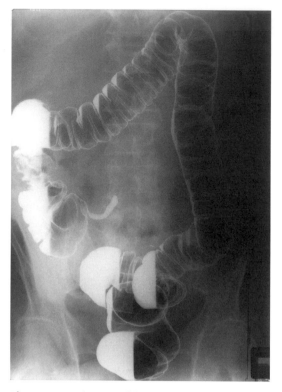

Fig. 4.43 Carcinoma of the ascending colon.

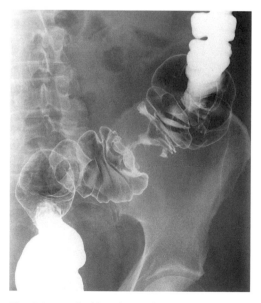

Fig. 4.44 Typical 'apple core' carcinoma in the sigmoid colon.

COLONIC CARCINOMA

Carcinoma of the colon, usually an adenocarcinoma, is the commonest malignancy of the intestinal tract, with the preponderance of lesions occurring in the rectosigmoid region. Predisposing factors include hereditary polyposis syndromes, chronic inflammatory bowel disease, family history of colonic carcinoma and possibly dietary causes.

RADIOLOGICAL INVESTIGATIONS

- Chest X-ray.
- Plain abdominal films.
- Barium enema or (colonoscopy).
- Intravenous urography (IVU) if there is suspected ureteric involvement.
- Ultrasound for liver metastases.
- CT/MRI for staging and pre-operative work-up.

RADIOLOGICAL FEATURES

Barium enema may demonstrate a malignant polyp. Features of more advanced tumours are:

- Annular carcinoma: predominantly infiltrates the bowel wall circumferentially causing irregular luminal narrowing with an 'apple-core' deformity. Overhanging edges cause a 'shouldering' defect.
- Polypoidal mass: produces an intraluminal filling defect, most commonly in the caecum.

COMPLICATIONS

- Obstruction: sometimes a presenting feature. Plain abdominal films may localize the level of obstruction. In equivocal cases, water-soluble contrast enema readily defines the site of obstruction prior to surgery.
- Perforation: secondary to bowel distension caused by tumour obstruction, may present with peritonitis.
- Fistula formation: from malignant infiltration of adjacent structures.

DIFFERENTIAL DIAGNOSIS OF COLONIC NARROWING

- Diverticular disease: usually in sigmoid colon.
- Crohn's disease: strictures may be single or multiple.
- Ulcerative colitis: benign or malignant strictures develop after prolonged bowel involvement.
- Extrinsic: inflammatory or neoplastic infiltration.
- Radiotherapy.
- Tuberculosis.
- Ischaemia.

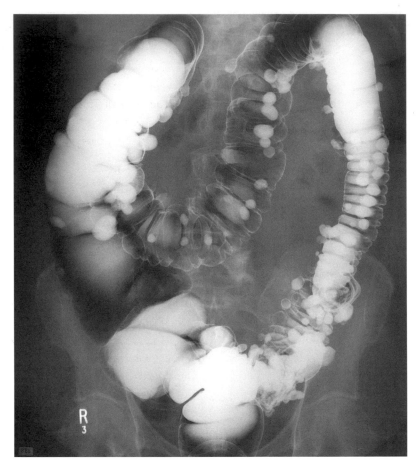

Fig. 4.45 Barium enema showing extensive diverticular disease throughout the colon.

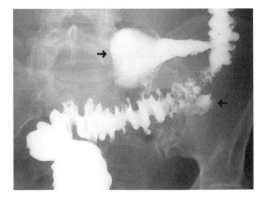

Fig. 4.46 Abscess formation (arrows) resulting from diverticular disease.

DIVERTICULAR DISEASE

Diverticular disease is a common disorder with colonic smooth-muscle hypertrophy associated with pouch-like protrusions between the thickened muscle fibres. There is herniation of the mucosa and submucosa through sites of weakness in the bowel wall. The sigmoid is the most frequently affected (>90%) but diverticula may arise from any part of the colon. A low-fibre diet is likely to be one aetiology of this condition.

RADIOLOGICAL INVESTIGATIONS

- Barium enema.
- Ultrasound, CT and mesenteric angiography for complications.

RADIOLOGICAL FEATURES

Barium enema examination will readily demonstrate the outpouchings as smooth round projections from the bowel wall. Diverticula vary considerably in size, from being just visible, to oval or round sacs several centimetres in diameter. Barium may persist in the diverticula for several weeks as there is no mechanism for emptying. The sigmoid colon may be narrow and irregular, and sometimes the appearances are very difficult to distinguish from a carcinoma.

COMPLICATIONS

- Diverticulitis: inflammatory changes leading to attacks of abdominal pain and fever.
- Pericolic abscess: perforation of a diverticulum often results in a localized pericolic abscess. A barium enema may show a sinus track leading from the sigmoid into the abscess. Ultrasound or CT may demonstrate the localized collection, which can sometimes be drained percutaneously.
- Perforation: free perforation of the diverticulum or abscess into the peritoneal cavity can give rise to a faecal peritonitis.
- Fistula formation: may result from rupture of an abscess or inflamed diverticulum into an adjacent organ, the commonest being the bladder (vesicocolic fistula), with pneumaturia as a presenting symptom. Fistulae may lead into the vagina, ureter, small bowel, colon or skin.
- Haemorrhage: probably from erosion of a bowel-wall artery, often from a right-colon diverticulum. Bleeding can be profuse and mesenteric angiography may localize the exact site of bleeding.

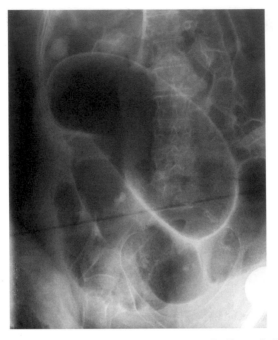

Fig. 4.47 Sigmoid volvulus with a grossly distended sigmoid.

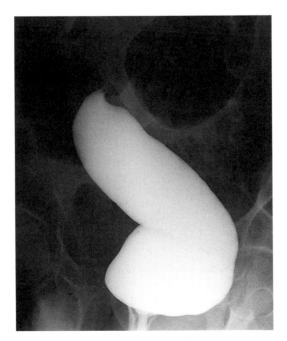

Fig. 4.48 Barium enema demonstrating the typical 'bird's beak' appearance at the site of obstruction in sigmoid volvulus.

VOLVULUS

Volvulus is the twisting of a segment of gut with subsequent obstruction.

Torsion refers to twisting without obstruction. The stomach, small bowel, caecum and sigmoid can all be involved, but the sigmoid is the most frequently affected.

Gastric volvulus. Rotation of the stomach occurs in either the vertical or organo-axial plane (line from pylorus to cardia).

Small-bowel volvulus. Mesenteric anomalies with a mobile bowel allow abnormal rotation and twisting, resulting in mechanical obstruction with possible vascular compromise.

Caecal volvulus. The caecum twists on its long axis. The distended gas-filled caecum is characteristically displaced upwards and into the left upper quadrant, with an empty right iliac fossa. The distal colon is devoid of air and growing caecal dilatation leads to a threat of perforation.

Sigmoid volvulus

Elderly and long-term psychiatric patients are particularly prone to this condition. Sigmoid volvulus occurs when there is rotation of the sigmoid about its axis, especially in a long redundant loop, to give rise to a closed-loop obstruction. Unrelieved obstruction may lead to vascular compromise, bowel infarction, or perforation.

RADIOLOGICAL FEATURES

The sigmoid loop can become very dilated to occupy the whole of the abdomen. It has the appearance of an inverted U with three dense lines, two lateral walls and a central line produced by the two adjacent inner walls, all converging into the large bowel mesenteric root in the pelvis. A barium enema demonstrates obstruction at the level of the volvulus, with the lumen of the bowel tapering to give a 'bird's beak' appearance.

TREATMENT

Decompression via a rectal tube through the twisted segment. A high recurrence rate of up to 80% often requires surgical resection of the redundant loop.

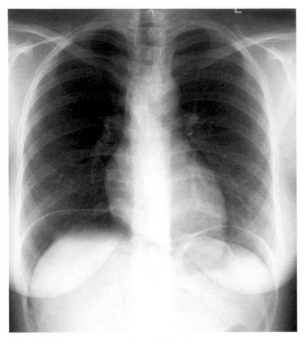

Fig. 4.49 Free gas under both diaphragms.

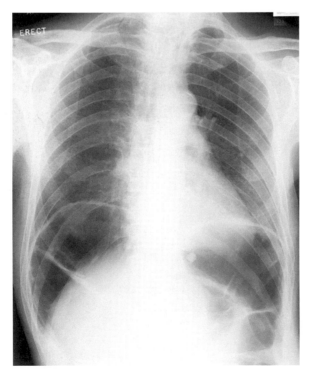

Fig. 4.50 Chilaiditi's syndrome: interposition of colon between diaphragm and liver or spleen.

AIR UNDER THE DIAPHRAGM

Free abdominal air is also referred to as 'pneumoperitoneum'.

• It accumulates under one or both diaphragms when the patient is erect.

• Even small quantities can be detected on plain films.

• The erect position has to be maintained for a few minutes before air can be visualized as a crescentic area of lucency between the right diaphragm and liver or left diaphragm and spleen.

• Lateral decubitus abdominal films can be used for very ill patients. The best projection is the left lateral decubitus when free air will be seen between the right lateral margin of the liver and the peritoneal surface.

• Free air will not be seen in up to 20–30% of patients.

CAUSES

• Post laparotomy or laparoscopy is the commonest cause.

• Viscus perforation (peptic ulcer, colonic diverticulum).

Sometimes difficulty is encountered identifying the free air, either because of viscus distension or confusing gas shadows below the diaphragm. Large-bowel interposition between the diaphragm and liver or spleen may simulate free air (Chilaiditi's syndrome).

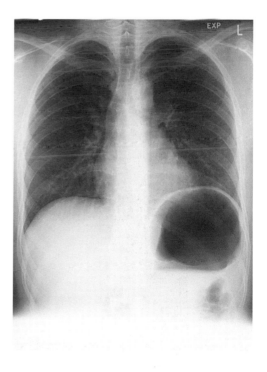

Fig. 4.51 Gas distension of the stomach; a common, normal finding.

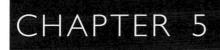

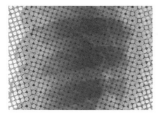

Liver and Pancreas

LIVER AND PANCREAS: INVESTIGATIONS

PLAIN FILMS

Aids detection of opaque gallbladder calculi, calcification in the gallbladder wall, gas in the biliary tree and pancreatic calcification.

ORAL CHOLECYSTOGRAM

An iodine-based oral contrast medium is ingested the evening before the examination. Films of the right upper quadrant the following day demonstrate an opacified gallbladder. It does not opacify if there is cystic duct obstruction or the patient is jaundiced. Calculi are seen as filling defects; a film after a fatty meal shows the extent of gall-bladder contraction.

OPERATIVE CHOLANGIOGRAM

This investigation is performed at cholecystectomy when the cystic duct is cannulated and contrast injected to outline the common bile duct. Exclusion of common bile duct stones avoids the need for surgical exploration.

T-TUBE CHOLANGIOGRAM

The examination may be carried out approximately 10 days after surgery to identify any remaining calculi in the common bile duct. Contrast is injected into the T-tube under fluoroscopic control to exclude residual calculi.

TRANSHEPATIC CHOLANGIOGRAM

A fine needle is inserted directly into a bile duct in the liver under local anaesthetic. Contrast is injected to visualize the entire biliary system and thus try and elucidate a cause for obstructive jaundice.

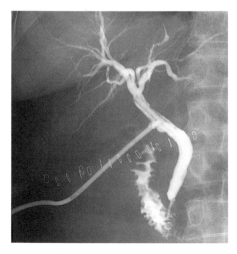 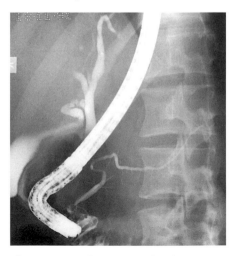

Fig. 5.1 Normal T-tube cholangiogram.

Fig. 5.2 Normal ERCP examination showing the pancreatic and common bile ducts.

ERCP

After the patient is sedated and the pharynx anaesthetized, an endoscope is introduced and advanced through the mouth into the duodenum, with cannulation and contrast injection into the ampulla of Vater, to demonstrate both the bile ducts and the pancreatic duct. Common bile duct stones can be removed through the endoscope by insertion of a catheter with a basket or balloon. Malignant common bile duct strictures can also be stented.

ULTRASOUND

• Liver ultrasound: the best basic imaging modality for focal or diffuse disease of the liver, staging primary tumours, detecting secondary deposits, investigation of calculi and jaundice and as an aid to liver biopsy or interventional procedures. Ultrasound will visualize the gallbladder, common bile duct, hepatic and portal veins.

• Pancreatic ultrasound: useful for suspected pancreatitis or tumour and to assist pancreatic biopsy.

ISOTOPE SCANNING (99m-technetium HIDA)

The isotope is accumulated by hepatocytes with excretion in bile. After a short transit time in the liver, the isotope is identified in the gallbladder and bile ducts at 15–20 minutes. Bowel activity is generally seen within an hour of injection. Excretion is severely delayed in biliary obstruction.

COMPUTED TOMOGRAPHY (CT)

Ultrasound is the first line of investigation, but if unsuccessful, CT is indicated. It demonstrates the full range of liver and pancreatic disease, including cirrhosis, tumours, pancreatitis and pancreatic carcinoma.

MAGNETIC RESONANCE IMAGING (MRI)

Provides excellent cross-sectional imaging as does CT, but without the risk of radiation. Blood vessels and bile ducts may be shown without injected contrast by using magnetic resonance angiography and magnetic resonance cholangiography.

ANGIOGRAPHY

Pre-operative assessment for the resection of pancreatic and liver tumours; vascular anatomy in portal hypertension.

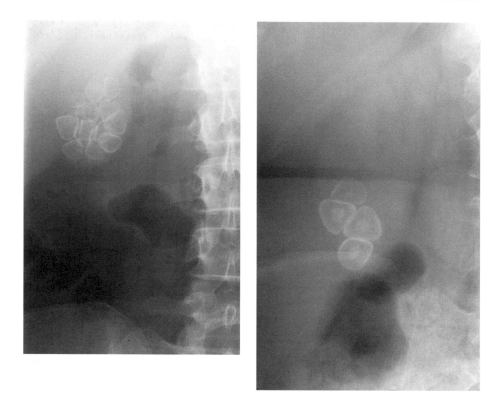

Fig. 5.3 Typical appearances of opaque gallbladder calculi on plain films.

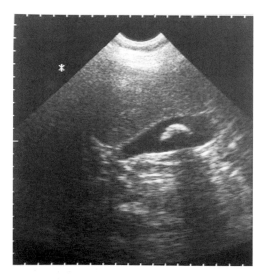

Fig. 5.4 Ultrasound of the gallbladder demonstrating a large single calculus. Note the acoustic shadow posterior to the gallstone.

GALLSTONES

Gallstones are common and occur in approximately 10% of the population with a marked female: male preponderance (4 : 1). There are three main types: mixed, cholesterol and pigment stones. Predisposing causes include obesity, diabetes, Crohn's disease, cirrhosis, pregnancy and haemolytic disease (sickle cell, thalassaemia).

RADIOLOGICAL FEATURES

• *Plain films* visualize approximately 10% of calculi as they are radiopaque. They may be faceted with multiple laminations.

• *Ultrasound* is the definitive investigation, where gallstones appear as echogenic areas casting a shadow. Gallbladder wall thickening and diameter of the common bile duct can also be assessed. Common bile duct stones are generally not accurately identified.

• *Cholecystography* is not now widely utilized but may assess function of the gallbladder.

COMPLICATIONS

• Acute cholecystitis: usually precipitated by obstruction of the cystic duct from a calculus.

• Chronic cholecystitis: chronic inflammation results in thickening and fibrosis of the gallbladder; it is frequently shrunken, and non-functioning.

• Biliary tract obstruction: secondary to the passage of a calculus into the common bile duct (choledocholithiasis) with obstructive jaundice.

• Acute pancreatitis: a strong association exists with gallstones. A stone at the lower end of the common bile duct not only impairs pancreatic drainage, but also promotes bile reflux into the pancreatic duct.

• Gallstone ileus: occurs when a gallstone ulcerates into the duodenum via a fistula and causes small bowel obstruction by stone impaction.

• Gallbladder carcinoma: rare, but usually associated with gallbladder calculi.

• Empyema: after a gallstone becomes wedged in the cystic duct, there is subsequent distension and inflammation, with purulent material filling the gallbladder.

TREATMENT

• Cholecystectomy or possible dissolution therapy/lithotripsy if unfit for surgery.

• ERCP for common bile duct calculi: sphincterotomy with basket or balloon removal of the stone.

• Empyema can be drained percutaneously under ultrasound control.

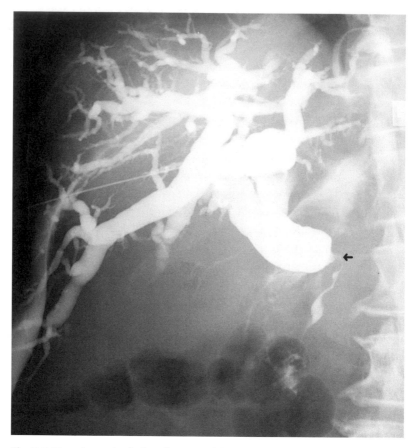

Fig. 5.5 Transhepatic cholangiogram: tight stricture from pancreatic carcinoma (arrow) causing severe biliary obstruction.

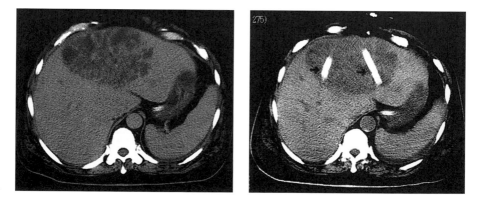

Fig. 5.6 Liver abscess: CT scans demonstrating a large low density lesion in the liver and after percutaneous insertion of drains (arrows).

COMMON BILE DUCT STRICTURE

Common bile duct narrowing is caused by numerous disorders resulting in biliary tract obstruction. The presenting features may be jaundice, fever and rigors (Charcot's triad).

RADIOLOGICAL FEATURES

- *Ultrasound* is the initial investigation of choice in a patient with jaundice. This may demonstrate a dilated common bile duct down to the level of the stricture.
- *ERCP* will show abnormalities of the upper gastrointestinal tract and the pancreas, in addition to the common bile duct stricture.
- *Transhepatic cholangiography* may be required if ERCP is unsuccessful.

CAUSES

Carcinoma of pancreas; chronic pancreatitis; postoperative; cholangiocarcinoma.

LIVER ABSCESS

A liver abscess is a localized collection of pus, which commonly results from cholangitis secondary to biliary tract obstruction. It may also follow suppurative inflammation in the drainage area of the portal vein in portal pyaemia. The latter may arise from inflammatory bowel disease, diverticulitis, appendicitis or a perforated viscus.

RADIOLOGICAL FEATURES

Ultrasound may show a single or multiple cavitating lesions. Abscesses are more common in the right lobe and on CT appear as low-density lesions, often showing peripheral ring-like enhancement after intravenous contrast. Occasionally, gas is seen centrally in the liver lesion, making the diagnosis of abscess certain. Hepatomegaly, elevation of the right diaphragm, pleural effusion and lower-lobe atelectasis may all be associated.

TREATMENT

- Antibiotics.
- Percutaneous drainage: abscesses can be drained under CT, ultrasound or fluoroscopic control.
- Surgical drainage.

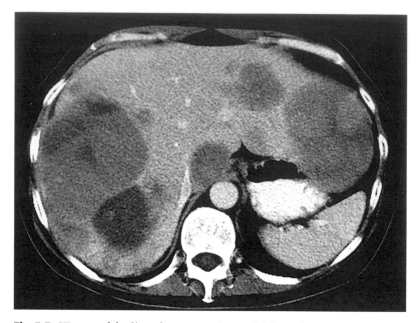

Fig. 5.7 CT scan of the liver demonstrating multiple well-defined metastases of different densities.

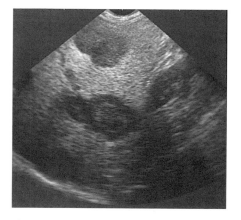
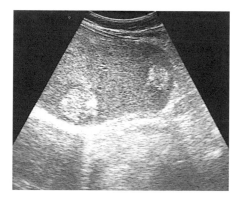

Fig. 5.8 Ultrasound of the liver; low and high echo metastases.

LIVER METASTASES

The liver is the most common organ as a site of secondary deposits. The most frequent neoplasms to metastasize to liver are those of colon, stomach, pancreas, breast and lung. Secondary deposits are much more common than primary liver tumours.

PRESENTATION

- Asymptomatic.
- Hepatomegaly.
- Ascites.
- Weight loss.
- Abnormal liver enzymes and jaundice
- Pre-operative check prior to surgery for primary carcinoma.
- Follow-up of primary carcinoma.

RADIOLOGICAL INVESTIGATION

- Plain films.
- Ultrasound.
- CT/MRI.
- Arteriography.
- Percutaneous biopsy (guided by ultrasound or CT).

RADIOLOGICAL FEATURES

- *Plain films* are usually not contributory. They may show hepatomegaly and occasionally calcified liver metastases.
- *Ultrasound* has a high degree of accuracy, and in a good quality study, is a very sensitive examination for the detection of metastases. The normal liver has a smooth outline with a homogeneous echo pattern. The essential feature of ultrasound is to demonstrate an abnormal echo pattern in the liver, metastases often being echo-poor, cystic, hyperechoic or diffusely infiltrative.
- *CT and MRI* are equally precise at detecting secondary deposits.
- *Arteriography* is only utilized in equivocal or difficult cases. Metastases are usually avascular but renal, melanoma, carcinoid and choriocarcinoma deposits tend to be vascular. Chemotherapy or embolization may be undertaken directly via the hepatic artery.

DIFFERENTIAL DIAGNOSIS

Haemangioma (common); hepatoma; abscess; haematoma.

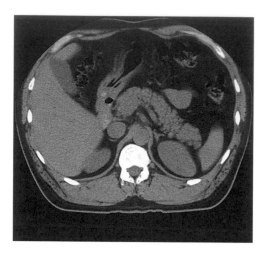

Fig. 5.9 CT scan of a normal pancreas.

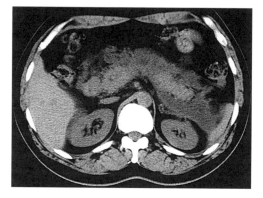

Fig. 5.10 Acute pancreatitis: CT scan showing inflammatory exudate surrounding the pancreas.

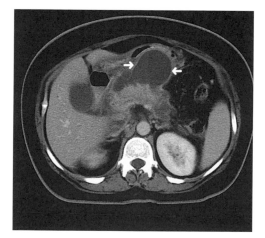

Fig. 5.11 CT scan showing a well-defined, low-density, pseudocyst (arrows).

ACUTE PANCREATITIS

Acute pancreatitis, an inflammatory condition of the pancreas has many aetiologies, but gallstones and alcohol abuse account for the vast majority. Mumps, certain drugs, surgical trauma and pancreatic carcinoma are some of the precipitating causes. Pancreatic function and morphology usually return to normal after an acute attack.

RADIOLOGICAL FEATURES

A plain chest X-ray often reveals pleural effusions (high amylase content); these are more common on the left side. An abdominal film may show gallstones, absence of gas in the abdomen (gasless abdomen) or an ileus. A 'sentinel loop of bowel' may be seen in the peripancreatic region. Gut distension obscures detail on ultrasound examination but the following may be visualized: an enlarged pancreas with dilatation of the pancreatic duct; gallstones; formation of pseudocysts; abscess; dilatation of common bile duct.

When an ultrasound examination is inadequate, CT is accurate in delineating the enlarged oedematous pancreas and its complications such as necrosis, haemorrhage and fluid collections. Contrast enhancement helps the surgeon by indicating the remaining viable organ. Serial CT follows the evolution of the inflammatory process.

COMPLICATIONS

- Pleural effusions and basal atelectasis.
- Necrotizing pancreatitis: proteolytic destruction of pancreatic parenchyma, with necrosis of the pancreas and surrounding fat, resulting in a solid inflammatory pancreatic mass called a 'phlegmon'. A high mortality rate is to be expected when this complication arises.
- Pancreatic ascites: due to perforation of the pancreatic duct.
- Jaundice from compression of the lower end of the common bile duct by the oedematous pancreas or by common bile duct calculi.
- Abscess: occurs after an acute attack, when a collection of necrotic pancreatic tissue becomes infected.
- Pseudocyst formation: results from escape of pancreatic secretions from the pancreatic duct or exudation from the surface of the inflamed pancreas; the lesser sac is the commonest location.
- Hypocalcaemia.
- Hyperglycaemia.

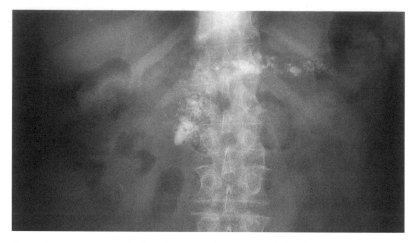

Fig. 5.12 Pancreatic calcification on a plain upper abdominal film.

Fig. 5.13 CT scan: pancreatic calcification (arrows).

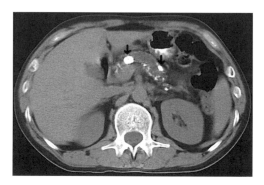

Fig. 5.14 ERCP: dilated irregular pancreatic duct in chronic pancreatitis.

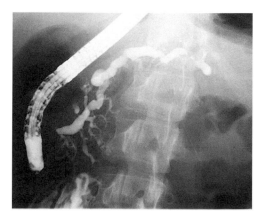

CHRONIC PANCREATITIS

Chronic pancreatitis is most commonly caused by alcohol abuse. The basic pathology is ductal stenosis and obstruction resulting in atrophy and fibrosis of the pancreas; irreversible damage to the pancreas results in abnormal pancreatic morphology. Gallstones are frequently associated with chronic pancreatitis.

PRESENTATION

Intermittent abdominal pain; weight loss; diarrhoea; steatorrhoea; jaundice; diabetes;

RADIOLOGICAL FEATURES

• Pancreatic calcification on abdominal X-ray or CT is virtually pathognomonic of chronic pancreatitis. Calcification is noted in approximately 50%, CT being more accurate in its detection, than a plain abdominal X-ray. Almost all calcification is intraductal, and it may be either diffusely spread or localized to a specific region.

• *Ultrasound and CT* may show a small, irregular atrophic pancreas with altered parenchymal pattern. Ascites may be associated.

• *ERCP* with cannulation and injection of contrast into the pancreatic duct may show an irregular dilated duct with stenoses, obstruction and non-filling of the side branches. Pseudocysts may fill if they communicate.

• *MRI* shows loss of signal intensity on T1 sequence.

COMPLICATIONS

• Jaundice from bile duct obstruction.
• Pseudocyst formation.
• Splenic, portal or mesenteric vein thrombosis.
• Malabsorption.

TREATMENT

• Medical: correcting diabetes and malabsorption by diet, insulin and pancreatic supplements.
• Surgical: cholecystectomy for gallstones; intervention for complications such as biliary obstruction or pseudocyst formation; partial or total pancreatectomy with drainage procedure of pancreatic duct. Cysts may be drained into the stomach under radiological guidance.

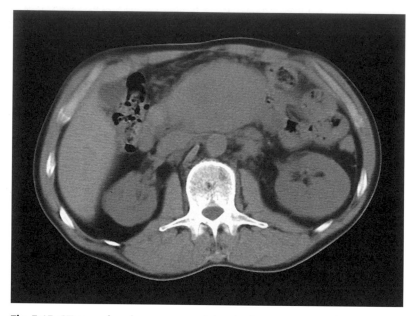

Fig. 5.15 CT scan showing an upper abdominal mass: pancreatic carcinoma.

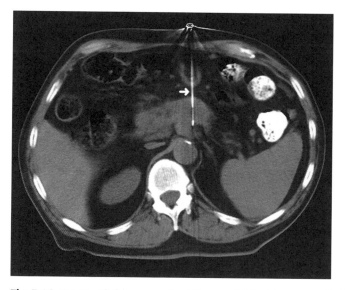

Fig. 5.16 Pancreatic biopsy under CT control. The biopsy needle has been inserted directly through the anterior abdominal wall (arrow).

PANCREATIC CARCINOMA

Pancreatic carcinoma is the fourth commonest malignant tumour after lung, colon and breast tumours. The most frequent pathological type arises from the pancreatic duct epithelium (adenocarcinoma). Tumours of the body and tail tend to be larger at the time of presentation. There is a very poor 5 year survival rate. Islet cell tumours such as insulinoma and glucagonoma are much less common and less aggressive.

PRESENTATION

Clinical symptoms usually occur late and at the time of presentation there is often local invasion of blood vessels or bowel. Only a small percentage of patients have the tumour confined to the pancreas, though peri-ampullary cancers may be localized.

- Abdominal pain, sometimes severe and continuous.
- Weight loss, anorexia.
- Obstructive jaundice.
- Malabsorption, diarrhoea.
- Diabetes.

RADIOLOGICAL FEATURES

- *Ultrasound* may demonstrate pancreatic and bile duct dilatation, a distended gallbladder, focal pancreatic enlargement with a hypo-echoic mass, liver metastases or ascites.
- *CT* will show similar findings and it may be more precise. CT may demonstrate local invasion into the retroperitoneal structures and metastases to the porta hepatis or the liver. A definitive diagnosis can often be obtained by a fine-needle or tru-cut biopsy of the mass.
- *MRI*: reduced signal from the pancreas on T1 sequence.
- *ERCP* is useful when ultrasound and CT are equivocal and may show an irregular ductal obstruction or vessel encasement.
- *Arteriography* is sometimes utilized to define the vascular anatomy prior to surgery.

TREATMENT

Local extension beyond the confines of the organ, invasion of adjacent structures such as stomach, and secondary deposits in the liver or ascites, usually render the tumour inoperable; only 10–15% are suitable for attempted curative resection; palliative surgical procedures for relief of jaundice; stenting via ERCP, or if this is not possible then percutaneous insertion; pancreaticoduodenectomy (Whipple's operation) for small periampullary lesions.

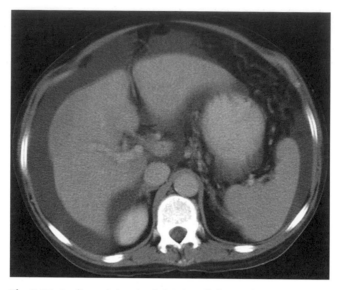

Fig. 5.17 Ascites: abdominal CT visualizing ascites as low density surrounding the liver and spleen.

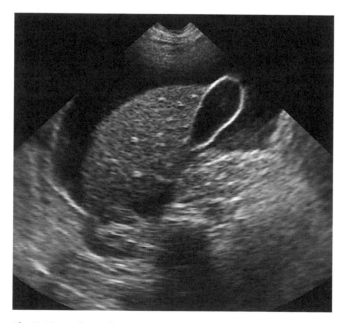

Fig. 5.18 Ascites: ultrasound examination demonstrates the free intra-abdominal collection (black) surrounding the liver and gallbladder.

ASCITES

Ascites refers to an accumulation of fluid within the abdominal cavity: in the supine position it collects in the most dependent parts, the pelvis and paracolic gutters.

• Haemorrhagic ascites: this suggests malignant involvement of peritoneum, though it may represent haemorrhage after trauma or liver biopsy.

• Chylous ascites: chyle may rarely accumulate in the peritoneal cavity. Causes include congenital lymphangiectasia, abdominal trauma including surgery with damage to abdominal lymphatic channels, malignant infiltration, filariasis and tuberculosis.

RADIOLOGICAL FEATURES

• *Plain abdomen films* may show generalized haziness of the abdomen, with loss of psoas outlines. Any gas containing small bowel loops float centrally.

• *Ultrasound* localizes fluid collections in the abdomen with considerable accuracy. The fluid appears anechoic, is freely mobile and bowel loops may be seen floating in the fluid. It can be aspirated, under ultrasound control, for a diagnostic tap or percutaneous drainage by means of a catheter can be undertaken.

• *CT* demonstrates ascites as a low-density margin around the intra-abdominal organs and is most clearly seen adjacent to the liver.

CAUSES

Transudate. Freely mobile, simple fluid collection.
• Cirrhosis.
• Hypoproteinaemia.
• Renal failure.
• Pericarditis.
• Cardiac failure.
• Budd–Chiari syndrome.

Exudate. Complex fluid collection and may contain solid tissue or inflammatory debris.
• Primary or secondary carcinoma.
• Tuberculous peritonitis.
• Pancreatitis.
• Meig's syndrome.

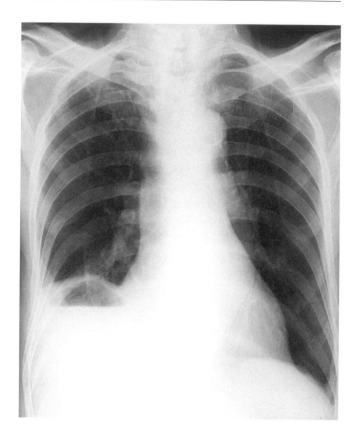

Fig. 5.19 Air/fluid level below the right diaphragm in subphrenic abscess.

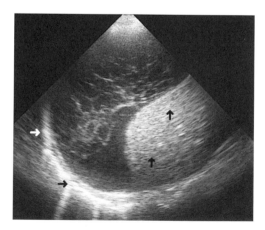

Fig. 5.20 Ultrasound reveals the abscess with multiple septations between the diaphragm (➜) and liver (↑).

SUBPHRENIC ABSCESS

A subphrenic abscess is a fluid collection between the diaphragm and the liver or spleen. It is a recognized complication of upper abdominal surgery but may occur as a result of perforation of the gastrointestinal tract. The abscess occurs more commonly on the right.

PRESENTATION

- Upper abdominal pain; shoulder pain; pyrexia (swinging).

RADIOLOGICAL INVESTIGATIONS

- Plain abdomen or chest film.
- Ultrasound.
- CT.
- Isotope scanning

RADIOLOGICAL FEATURES

- *Plain chest films* may feature a pleural effusion or basal collapse and consolidation. An elevated diaphragm on the affected side and a gas or fluid level under the diaphragm are diagnostic features.
- *Ultrasound and CT* will demonstrate the volume and extent of the collection.
- *Isotope scanning* with Indium-labelled white cells, shows increased activity at the site of the abscess, but is rarely necessary for diagnosis.

TREATMENT

- Percutaneous drainage either under ultrasound or CT guidance.
- Surgical drainage.

OTHER SITES OF ABDOMINAL ABSCESS FORMATION

- Psoas abscess: commonly tuberculous but may be pyogenic.
- Pancreatic abscess: follows acute pancreatitis.
- Renal/perinephric abscess: often haematogenous spread or secondary to renal obstruction; diabetics are particularly susceptible.
- Pelvic abscess: results in diarrhoea due to rectal irritation and inflammation.
- Liver abscess: pyogenic or amoebic.
- Appendix abscess: perforation of the appendix may lead to a localized abscess. An abdominal X-ray may show a calcified appendicolith.
- Pericolic abscess: particularly from diverticular disease.
- Intra-abdominal abscess: secondary to bowel perforation.

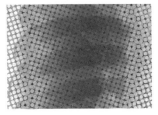

CHAPTER 6

Urinary Tract

THE URINARY TRACT: INVESTIGATIONS

PLAIN FILMS

A plain abdominal film is essential prior to urinary tract investigation. This may show: renal calculi in the pelvicalyceal system, renal parenchymal calcification, ureteric calculi, bladder calcification and calculi, prostatic calcification or sclerotic bone deposits.

Caution should be used in interpreting renal-tract calcification as overlying calcified mesenteric glands and pelvic vein phleboliths are often mistaken for ureteric calculi. Inspiration and expiration films change the position of the kidneys and often confirm that a calcified area in the upper abdomen is a calculus.

INTRAVENOUS UROGRAPHY (IVU)

The indications for this examination are haematuria, renal calculi, ureteric colic or suspected calculi. Patients with urinary retention and urinary tract-infection should initially have an ultrasound rather than an IVU. Patient preparation:

• A laxative the day before the examination to clear gas and faecal shadowing from the abdomen so that the renal outlines are not obscured.

• Fluid restriction for 6–8 hours prior to the examination to increase concentration of the urine and produce a denser pyelogram. Patients in renal failure, and those with diabetes and multiple myeloma should not be dehydrated.

• Elicit a history of iodine allergy prior to intravenous injection and do not proceed if positive.

After a preliminary control film of the abdomen, 50–100 ml of a low osmolar iodinated contrast medium is injected. Contrast rapidly reaches the kidney and is excreted by glomerular filtration. A film taken shortly after injection demonstrates the nephrogram phase showing the renal parenchyma and outline. Films after 5, 10 and 15 minutes reveal contrast in the pelvicalyceal systems, ureters and bladder; the series is varied according to the individual patient. Renal obstruction may require a delayed study up to 24 hours to outline the pelvicalyceal system.

RETROGRADE PYELOGRAPHY

A retrograde pyelogram is occasionally necessary when detail of the pelvi-calyceal system and ureter is not adequately delineated by intravenous contrast, especially when there is suspicion of an epithelial tumour of the urinary tract. In theatre, a catheter is placed into the ureter after a cystoscopy; contrast injected through the catheter outlines the pelvicalyceal system and ureter.

MICTURATING CYSTOGRAM

A catheter is inserted in the bladder which is filled to capacity with contrast. After catheter removal, films are taken of the renal tract as the patient is micturating, looking for vesico-ureteric reflux. Careful examination of the urethra in the oblique position is necessary in suspected urethral valves, as they are usually only demonstrated during micturition.

ANTEGRADE PYELOGRAPHY

If for technical reasons, a retrograde pyelogram is not possible (e.g. after cystectomy), a fine-gauge needle, under local anaesthetic, can be inserted directly into the pelvicalyceal system and contrast injected to visualize the calyces, pelvis and ureter. The patient lies in a prone position and the examination is carried out under either ultrasound or fluoroscopic control. This procedure, not requiring a general anaesthetic, accurately localizes the site of an obstructing lesion, such as a calculus or stricture.

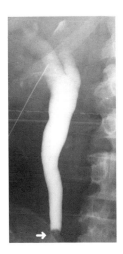

Fig. 6.1 Antegrade pyelogram showing ureteric obstruction by a non-opaque calculus (arrow).

PERCUTANEOUS NEPHROSTOMY

Provides temporary drainage of an obstructed kidney by percutaneous insertion of a catheter directly into the pelvicalyceal system.

URETHROGRAPHY

The adult male urethra can be visualised by:

• Ascending urethrography: contrast is injected into the meatus and films obtained of the urethra.

• Descending urethrography: after filling the bladder with contrast, the catheter is removed and films of the urethra are taken during micturition. In both studies, the entire urethra must be studied.

ULTRASOUND

Ultrasound is one of the most valuable investigations of the urinary tract and the investigation of choice in children. It is extremely effective in evaluating renal size, growth, masses, renal obstruction, bladder residual volumes and prostatic size; it is non-invasive and can be repeated frequently. Ultrasound probe technology has shown great recent advances and exact details can be obtained by the technique of endo-ultrasound — imaging after insertion of the probe in the rectum or vagina.

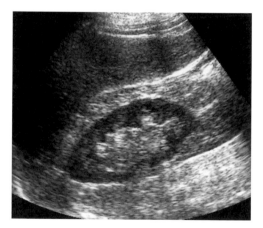

Fig. 6.2 Normal renal ultrasound.

COMPUTED TOMOGRAPHY (CT)

This aids assessment of renal masses, obstruction, retroperitoneal disease, staging of renal and bladder neoplasms, tumour invasion into the renal vein or inferior vena cava (IVC), and evaluation after trauma, surgery or chemotherapy.

ISOTOPES

• Static scanning: technetium-99m DMSA: selective uptake by the renal cells with stagnation in the proximal tubules produces images of the renal parenchyma. The isotope is used to assess function, position, size and scarring of kidneys.

• Dynamic scanning: technetium-99m DTPA: isotope clearance by glomerular filtration produces a dynamic scan, providing information on renal blood flow and renal function. The function of each individual kidney can be assessed as well as total renal function.

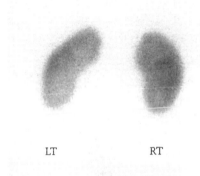

LT   RT

DIVIDED RENAL FUNCTION

%LT KIDNEY = 41.492

%RT KIDNEY = 58.508

Fig. 6.3 DMSA scan showing relative function of each kidney.

ARTERIOGRAPHY

Evaluation of the renal arterial circulation may be necessary for:

• further investigation of equivocal renal masses: renal cell carcinomas are usually hypervascular with a pathological circulation;

• arteriovenous malformation;

• renal artery stenosis;

• anatomical details prior to renal transplantation, or suspected vascular occlusion after surgery.

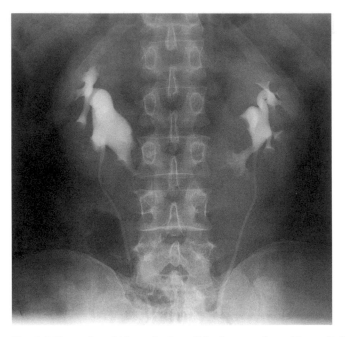

Fig. 6.4 Horseshoe kidney: fusion of the lower poles with medially pointing calyces.

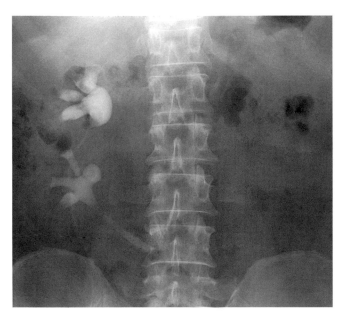

Fig. 6.5 Crossed renal ectopia.

CONGENITAL RENAL ANOMALIES

Unilateral renal agenesis. During urinary-tract investigations an incidental absence of a kidney may be discovered. Technetium-99m DMSA isotope scan will confirm this finding.

Renal hypoplasia. The kidney is small but perfectly formed.

Horseshoe kidney. Fusion of the opposite renal poles (usually the lower). There is an increased incidence of: pelvi-ureteric junction (PUJ) obstruction; renal calculi; infection.

Crossed fused renal ectopia. One kidney is displaced across the midline and fused to the other normal kidney; ureteric orifices lie in a normal position.

Pelvic kidney. May be associated with vesico-ureteric reflux and hydronephrosis due to an abnormal ureteric insertion.

Duplex kidney. The commonest renal anomaly with a variable degree of duplication ranging from minor changes of the renal pelvis, to total duplication of the renal pelvis and ureter.

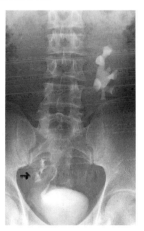

Fig. 6.7 Pelvic kidney (arrow).

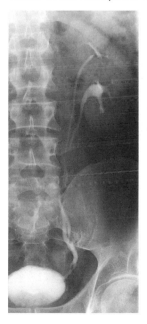

Fig. 6.6 Left duplex kidney; the ureters join in the pelvis.

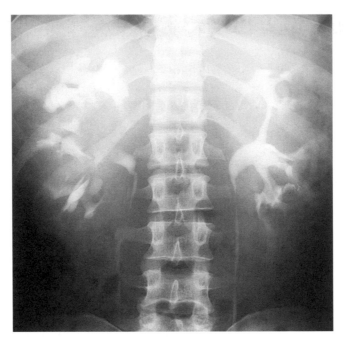

Fig. 6.8 Polycystic kidneys: IVU demonstrating enlarged kidneys with a distorted calyceal pattern.

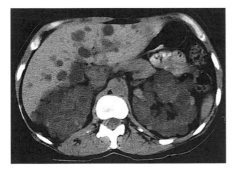

Fig. 6.9 CT abdomen: multiple cysts in the kidneys and liver.

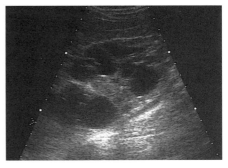

Fig. 6.10 Ultrasound: multiple renal cysts seen as low echo lesions.

POLYCYSTIC KIDNEYS

Polycystic kidneys are characterized by enlargement of both kidneys with replacement of normal renal tissue by multiple cysts. Expansion and enlargement of cysts compress the renal substance, leading to loss of function and eventually renal failure.

Polycystic disease of adults:	Inherited as an autosomal dominant with nearly 100% penetration.
Polycystic disease of childhood:	Presents at 3–5 years of age with enlarged kidneys and hepatic fibrosis. Death may result from portal hypertension.
Polycystic disease of the new-born:	Discovered in the first few days of life with renal failure and gross enlargement of both kidneys.

PRESENTATION

Manifestations of adult polycystic disease usually arise in the third and fourth decades. Haematuria; palpable abdominal mass; proteinuria; renal failure.

RADIOLOGICAL FEATURES

Renal enlargement is often of massive proportions.

• *Intravenous urography* may show elongation, deformity and distortion of the calyces. The renal pelvis may also be deformed by cysts protruding into it.

• *Ultrasound and CT* accurately measure the renal size and assess the number and distribution of cysts. The disease may be diagnosed antenatally by ultrasound.

• *Technetium 99m scanning* will assess renal function.

ASSOCIATED FEATURES/COMPLICATIONS

• Cysts in the liver, pancreas and spleen.

• Increased incidence of intracranial aneurysms. Rarely, polycystic disease may first manifest itself by signs and symptoms of a ruptured intracranial aneurysm (subarachnoid haemorrhage).

• Hypertension.

• Renal calculi.

• Urinary-tract infections.

• Uraemia: may eventually need dialysis or renal transplantation.

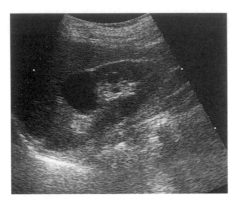

Fig. 6.11 Ultrasound: simple renal cyst.

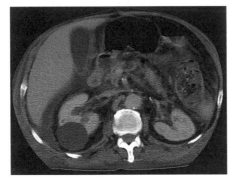

Fig. 6.12 CT showing a well-defined right renal cyst.

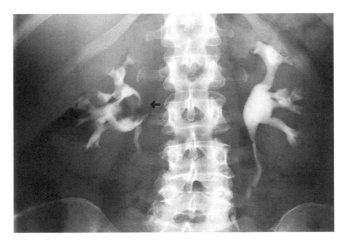

Fig. 6.13 Filling defect in the right renal pelvis (arrow), proved to be a transitional cell carcinoma.

RENAL CYST

Simple renal cysts are extremely common, occurring with increasing frequency as age progresses. They are often multiple, of varying size and usually an incidental finding. Renal cysts are almost always asymptomatic, of little clinical significance, and usually require no further treatment.

RADIOLOGICAL FEATURES

- *Intravenous pyelography*: cysts appear as mass lesions causing a bulge in the renal outline, often with pelvicalyceal distortion.
- *Ultrasound*: well defined with few or no internal echoes and transmission of the sound beam with posterior acoustic enhancement.
- *CT*: sharply delineated homogeneous lesions with no enhancement after intravenous contrast.
- *MRI*: well circumscribed low signal lesion (black) or a uniform high signal (white) depending on the type of sequence used (T1 or T2).

    Complicated cysts (haemorrhagic cysts, calcified cysts, cysts with internal septations) need follow up with possible needle aspiration for cytology or histology.

RENAL PELVIC/URETERIC TUMOURS

Tumours arising from the urinary tract epithelium are usually transitional cell carcinomas. They may be polypoidal, plaque-like or form strictures. Squamous cell carcinoma is often associated with either calculi or chronic infection such as schistosomiasis. Haematuria is the main presenting symptom.

RADIOLOGICAL FEATURES

The majority of urothelial tumours produce an intraluminal mass seen on intravenous urography as irregular filling defects, occasionally villous or lobulated. Ureteric tumours often exhibit a localized dilatation of the ureter at the site of the tumour, but sometimes antegrade or retrograde pyelography is necessary for further evaluation. Ureteroscopy with biopsy will confirm the findings.

Differential diagnosis of filling defect in ureter/renal pelvis

- Calculus.
- Blood clot.
- Tumour.
- Papillary necrosis (diabetes, analgesic abuse).

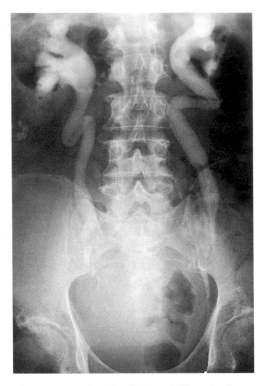

Fig. 6.14 IVU showing bilateral dilated calyces and ureters in bladder outlet obstruction.

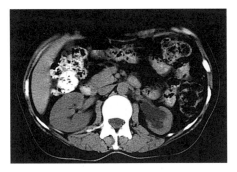

Fig. 6.15 CT scan: unrelieved obstruction leading to renal atrophy of the left kidney.

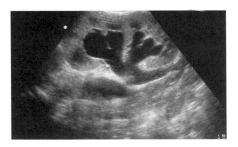

Fig. 6.16 Ultrasound: renal obstruction showing dilated calyces.

RENAL-TRACT OBSTRUCTION

Obstruction to the renal tract may occur at many sites: the pelvicalyceal system, ureter, bladder or bladder outlet. The commonest cause is a ureteric calculus but tumours of the urinary tract or extrinsic ureteric invasion from rectosigmoid or gynaecological tumours are also well-recognized causes. If left untreated, renal atrophic changes may follow.

RADIOLOGICAL FEATURES

The different imaging modalities all diagnose renal tract dilatation.

• *Ultrasound.* This is the initial investigation of choice. The distended collecting system is seen as an echo-free area in the centre of the kidney.

• *IVU.* Excretion of contrast is delayed with distended and clubbed calyces, often with ureteric dilatation down to the level of obstruction. Slow excretion of contrast may require delayed films up to 24 hours.

• *CT.* Demonstrates the distended collecting system and ureters as well as detecting extrinsic causes of obstruction, such as tumours.

• *Isotope scanning.* Identifies a slow accumulation and clearance of isotope in the collecting system.

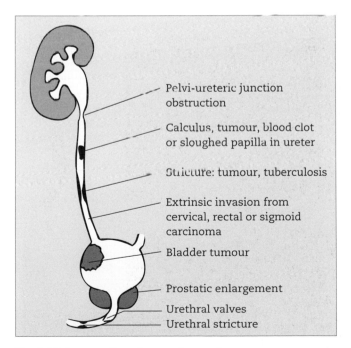

Pelvi-ureteric junction obstruction

Calculus, tumour, blood clot or sloughed papilla in ureter

Stricture: tumour, tuberculosis

Extrinsic invasion from cervical, rectal or sigmoid carcinoma

Bladder tumour

Prostatic enlargement

Urethral valves

Urethral stricture

Fig. 6.17 Causes of renal-tract obstruction.

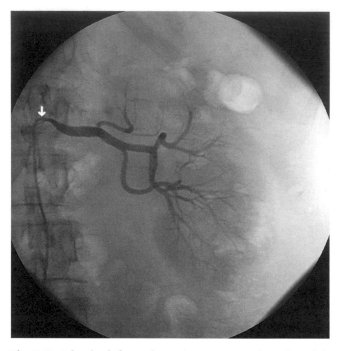

Fig. 6.18 Selective left renal arteriogram: stenosis at the origin of the left renal artery (arrow).

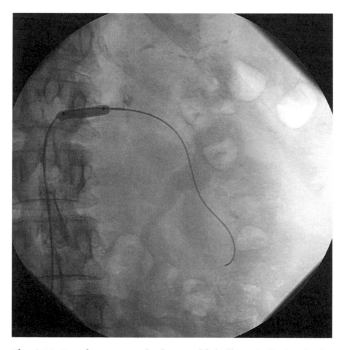

Fig. 6.19 Renal artery angioplasty with balloon inflation in the stenosis.

RENAL ARTERY STENOSIS

Renal artery stenosis results from a narrowing of the renal artery leading to reduction in perfusion pressure, hypertension and a decrease in renal size. It is usually atherosclerotic in nature and may be uni- or bilateral.

PRESENTATION

- Hypertension.
- Deteriorating renal function.

RADIOLOGICAL FEATURES

- *Ultrasound* may demonstrate a small kidney. A Doppler examination may show abnormal flow patterns in the renal artery with an increased peak systolic velocity.
- *Intravenous urography* is not reliable and may be entirely normal but classically the affected side shows:

    delayed appearance and a slow excretion of contrast medium;

    reduction in pole to pole diameter of $\geqslant 1.5$ cm;

    increased concentration of contrast medium in the pelvicalyceal system, because of greater salt and water reabsorption from a slower tubular passage.

- *Isotope scanning* does not accurately diagnose stenosis but may demonstrate a reduced uptake in the affected kidney, with a delay in peak concentration.
- *Renal arteriography* is the definitive investigation to show the narrowing, with selective catheterization, and contrast injection into the renal arteries. Stenoses may be due to:
- Atheroma: commonest cause with stenosis of the proximal artery.
- Fibromuscular hyperplasia: a condition of unknown aetiology, most commonly seen in young women. Irregular intimal hyperplasia gives rise to a beaded appearance with stenosis in the distal renal arteries.

TREATMENT

- Balloon angioplasty or insertion of metallic stents.
- Surgical reconstruction of the renal artery:

    vein patch graft;

    splenic artery revascularization;

    prosthetic by-pass graft.

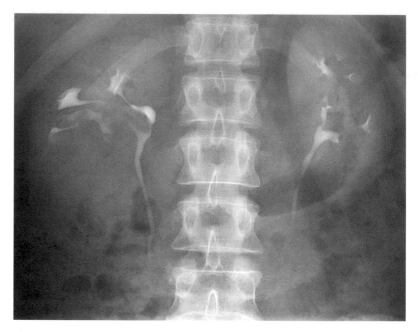

Fig. 6.20 IVU: mass in the lower pole of the right kidney causing calyceal distortion.

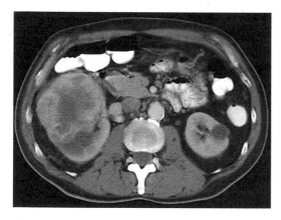

Fig. 6.21 Contrast enhanced CT: large right renal carcinoma. Note simple cyst in the left kidney.

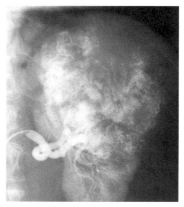

Fig. 6.22 Arteriogram demonstrating a pathological circulation in renal carcinoma.

RENAL CARCINOMA

Renal carcinoma arises from the renal tubular epithelium, an adenocarcinoma (hypernephroma) and up to 10% may be bilateral.

Wilms' tumour (nephroblastoma) is one of the more common malignancies occurring in children and these may also be bilateral in up to 10%.

Transitional cell carcinomas arise from the epithelium lining the pelvicalyceal system.

Secondary malignant infiltration of the kidneys may be occasionally encountered in lymphoma or leukaemia.

PRESENTATION

Pyrexia; haematuria; polycythaemia; first symptoms from secondary deposits to lung, bone, liver or brain such as haemoptysis, cough or pathological fractures; left varicocele if the left renal vein is occluded by tumour.

RADIOLOGICAL INVESTIGATION

Numerous investigations are available including plain films, intravenous urography; ultrasound; CT; MRI; arteriography and isotope bone scan (for secondary deposits).

RADIOLOGICAL FEATURES

• *Plain films*: occasionally show fine stippled or even curvilinear calcification in the renal mass.

• *Intravenous urography*: may reveal a soft-tissue mass causing a bulge in the renal outline, an enlargement of the kidney or pelvicalyceal distortion and irregularity. A large tumour may give rise to a completely non-functioning kidney.

• *Ultrasound*: highly accurate in distinguishing between a solid carcinoma and a benign cyst. Blood-flow characteristics of the renal tumour can be ascertained and in doubtful cases a biopsy taken under ultrasound control.

• *CT/MRI*: useful for staging to determine: calcification, size and density of the mass; perinephric tissue invasion; invasion into the renal veins and inferior vena cava; lymph-node enlargement.

• *Arteriography* is not often indicated but when utilized may demonstrate a pathological circulation in the vast majority of carcinomas.

DIFFERENTIAL DIAGNOSIS OF RENAL MASS

• Non-malignant: renal cysts, inflammatory masses, haematoma.

• Benign: adenoma, haemangioma, papilloma, angiomyolipoma.

• Malignant: renal cell carcinoma, transitional cell carcinoma, Wilms' tumour (nephroblastoma).

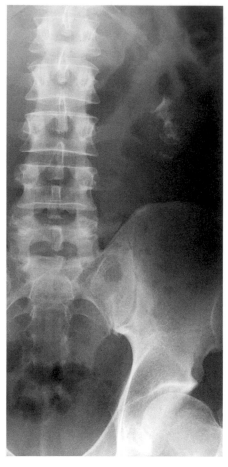

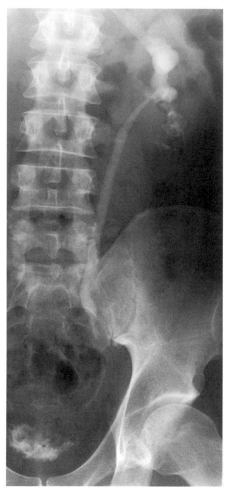

Fig. 6.23 Tuberculosis: plain film showing coarse calcification in the lower pole of the left kidney.

Fig. 6.24 IVU showing calyceal and ureteric dilatation due to a lower ureteric stricture.

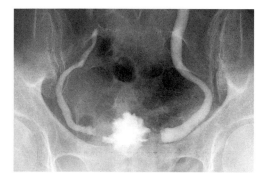

Fig 6.25 Contracted bladder in tuberculosis.

TUBERCULOSIS OF THE URINARY TRACT

After pulmonary tuberculosis, the renal tract is the most common site of infection, usually due to haematogenous spread either from pulmonary or bone tuberculosis. Any part of the renal tract may be involved: kidneys, ureters, bladder, seminal vesicles and epididymis.

RADIOLOGICAL FEATURES

A chest film should be performed to exclude pulmonary tuberculosis. Plain abdominal films may reveal calcification in the kidneys, seminal vesicles or vas deferens. Calcification is of a variable intensity, ranging from a few small flecks to heavy dense areas in advanced cases. Gross renal disorganization may lead to a non-functioning kidney (tuberculous autonephrectomy). Testicular ultrasound is useful to delineate epididymitis.

On IVU, the following features may be found.

• Kidneys: deformities of calyces, strictures, irregular cavity formation and scarring of renal parenchyma.

• Ureters: strictures and areas of narrowing in the ureters, the strictures often being multiple. Spread is usually from the kidneys, so renal abnormalities are often found.

• Bladder: tuberculous cystitis: initially there is mucosal oedema but subsequently bladder irregularity with contraction. The bladder has a thickened wall, is shrunken and of a small capacity.

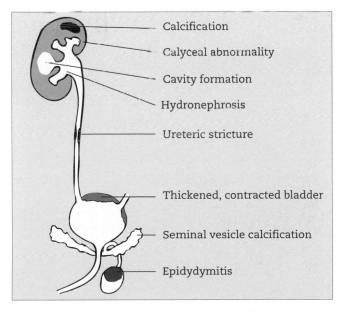

Calcification

Calyceal abnormality

Cavity formation

Hydronephrosis

Ureteric stricture

Thickened, contracted bladder

Seminal vesicle calcification

Epididymitis

Fig. 6.26 Manifestations of renal-tract tuberculosis.

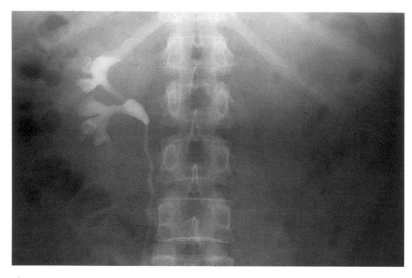

Fig. 6.27 IVU: non-visualization of the left kidney.

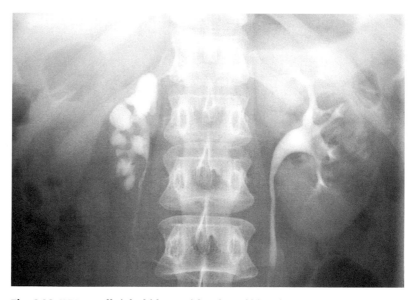

Fig. 6.28 IVU: small right kidney with calyceal blunting in chronic pyelonephritis.

UNILATERAL NON-FUNCTIONING KIDNEY

When one kidney is not visualized during intravenous pyelography, it may be absent, lying in an abnormal position, or grossly hydronephrotic. Numerous other causes of non-visualization of a kidney should also be considered. Ultrasound may demonstrate the size, position and degree of obstruction of a non-visualized kidney.

Isotope scanning may also be helpful as it will demonstrate the presence of an ectopic kidney.

CAUSES

• Chronic obstruction: ureteric obstruction from calculus, tumour or extrinsic invasion will lead to deterioration of function and atrophy.
• Vascular causes: renal artery occlusion either from severe atheromatous disease or following trauma; renal vein thrombosis.
• Tumour: renal carcinoma infiltrating the whole kidney.
• Chronic infection: chronic pyelonephritis, tuberculosis.
• Postnephrectomy.
• Renal agenesis.
• Ectopic kidney.

UNILATERAL SMALL KIDNEY

The normal kidney measures 9–14 cm in length, the left usually being larger than the right. However, a difference in size of >1.5 cm is regarded as significant.

CAUSES

• Chronic pyelonephritis: reduction in renal size, irregularity of outline due to focal areas of scarring and calyceal deformity. Scarring is most common in the upper pole of the kidney over the dilated calyces.
• Ischaemia: renal artery stenosis leading to decreased perfusion.
• Postobstructive atrophy: smooth outline, uniform loss of renal substance, with some dilatation of calyces. Severe obstruction, regardless of the cause, lasting longer than a few days may lead to irreversible loss of renal parenchyma and function, hence the importance of diagnosing and relieving renal-tract obstruction.
• Congenital hypoplasia: a small kidney with a smooth outline and a normal pelvicalyceal system.
• Renal infarction: here the scar is opposite a normal calyx.

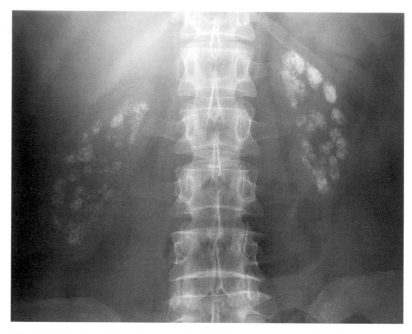

Fig. 6.29 Nephrocalcinosis: organized diffuse renal parenchymal calcification.

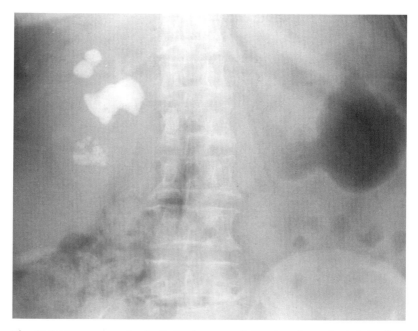

Fig. 6.30 Opaque renal calculi: the large medially placed opacity is lying in the renal pelvis.

NEPHROCALCINOSIS

'Nephrocalcinosis' refers to calcium deposition in the renal parenchyma, either in the cortex or medulla. The calcification is fairly uniform and may be a consequence of:

- Hypercalcaemia or hypercalcuria:
  hyperparathyroidism, usually primary; renal tubular acidosis; sarcoidosis; multiple myeloma.
- Structural renal abnormality:
  medullary sponge kidney—congenitally dilated tubules with deposition of calcium; papillary necrosis.

FOCAL RENAL PARENCHYMAL CALCIFICATION

- Tuberculosis: variable distribution of the renal calcification.
- Tumours: renal cell carcinoma.

RENAL CALCULUS

The majority of renal calculi are either pure oxalate, calcium oxalate, calcium oxalate with phosphate, uric acid or cystine. Predisposing factors:

Stasis due to congenital abnormalities (horseshoe kidney), pelvi-ureteric junction obstruction, renal-tract obstruction and ureterocele.

Metabolic causes: hyperparathyroidism; hypercalcuria; uric acid stones after cytotoxic therapy, gout, polycythaemia or after cytotoxic therapy; cystine stones in cystinuria.

Infection: typically *Proteus* infection, often resulting in staghorn calculi.

RADIOLOGICAL FEATURES

A plain abdominal film will generally reveal calculi as they are radio-opaque, except for uric acid stones which are radiolucent. The majority of calculi form in the calyces and may be seen on intravenous urography as a filling defect in the contrast column.

Staghorn calculi develop in the pelvicalyceal system and are usually easily visualized on plain films.

TREATMENT

- Extracorporeal lithotripsy (EL).
- Percutaneous removal under radiological control (nephrolithotomy).
- Surgery for large staghorn calculi or when EL and percutaneous approach has failed.

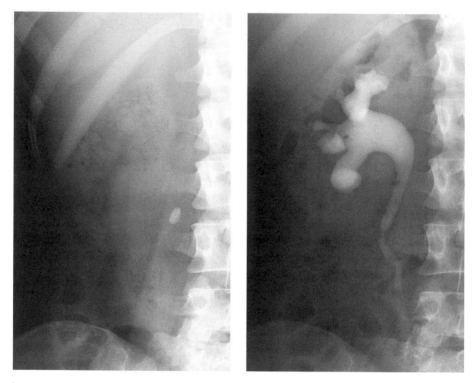

Fig. 6.31 Ureteric calculus: plain film and after IVU demonstrating obstruction.

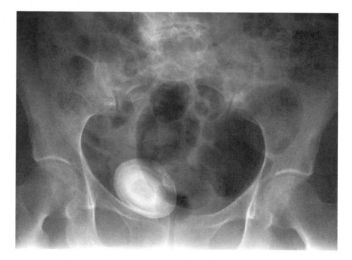

Fig. 6.32 Large opaque, laminated bladder calculus.

URETERIC CALCULUS

A ureteric calculus tends to be small, often 2–3 mm in diameter, and originates from the kidney. Its progress down the ureter may cause severe
abdominal pain; it commonly impacts at the vesico-ureteric junction.

RADIOLOGICAL FEATURES

A plain abdominal film may identify a small area of calcification in line with
the ureter. However, an intravenous urogram is required to confirm that
this opacity is a ureteric calculus, usually identified as a filling defect in the
contrast-filled ureter. If causing obstruction, there may be a delay in excretion of contrast, with a variable degree of pelvicalyceal distension and
ureteric dilatation to the level of the calculus. In severe obstruction, a temporary nephrostomy or double J ureteric stent may be needed.

TREATMENT

- Majority of calculi ≤5 mm in diameter pass spontaneously.
- Upper and lower third ureteric calculi: extracorporeal lithotripsy.
- Middle third: push calculus into renal pelvis and then lithotripsy.
- Lower third: endoscopic removal with a basket.
- Large calculi: may need open ureterotomy.

BLADDER CALCULUS

Calculi may descend from the kidney into the bladder or result from:
- urine infection, especially *Proteus*;
- urine stasis due to bladder outlet obstruction, bladder diverticulum or
neuropathic bladder;
- foreign bodies in the bladder.

RADIOLOGICAL FEATURES

Calculi may be missed on plain films due to overlying bony structures, gas
and faecal shadowing in the rectum, phleboliths or arterial calcification.
When the bladder is filled with contrast, either at IVU or cystography,
bladder stones may appear as filling defects. Ultrasound can also detect
them as echogenic structures casting an acoustic shadow.

TREATMENT

- Endoscopic removal with lithotrite.
- Large calculi may need open removal.
- Extracorporeal lithotripsy not widely used for bladder calculi.

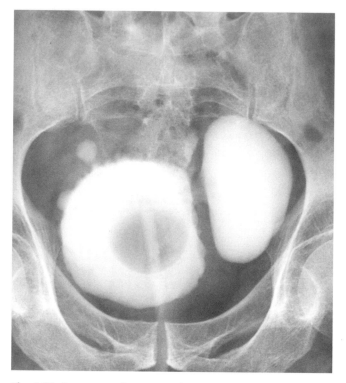

Fig. 6.33 Cystogram demonstrating a large left bladder diverticulum with further smaller diverticula on the right. An inflated balloon catheter is present in the bladder.

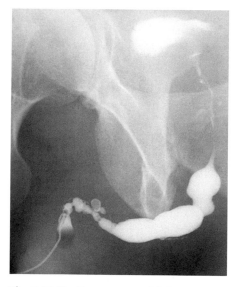

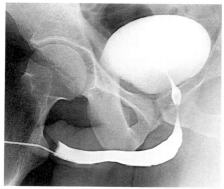

Fig. 6.35 Normal urethrogram. The smooth narrowing in the posterior and prostatic urethra is normal.

Fig. 6.34 Urethrogram: multiple strictures in the anterior urethra.

BLADDER DIVERTICULUM

A mucosal outpouching from the bladder muscle wall results in a bladder diverticulum. They may be:

- acquired secondary to lower urinary-tract obstruction or bladder instability;
- associated with a neurogenic bladder;
- congenital.

In males, the commonest cause of diverticula formation is a consequence of raised intravesical pressure with detrusor hypertrophy or from obstruction secondary to prostatic enlargement. Diverticula may be multiple and of a variable size, with some reaching enormous proportions.

IVU. Seen as outpouchings from the bladder wall.

Micturating cystography. Visualizes diverticula, especially during micturition when they distend; subsequent emptying of the diverticulum into the bladder at the end of micturition leaves a residual volume and may result in double micturition. Stasis leads to an increased incidence of calculus formation, urinary-tract infection and tumour. Residual urine volume in the bladder and diverticulum may be accurately measured by ultrasound.

URETHRAL STRICTURE

Strictures in the urethra are demonstrated by either a retrograde injection of contrast into the meatus (ascending urethrogram) or after instilling contrast into the bladder, obtaining films as the patient is micturating (descending urethrogram). Strictures present with symptoms of a slow urinary stream and outflow obstruction.

CAUSES

- Post trauma: following previous instrumentation, catheterization or external trauma. The strictures most commonly occur at the penoscrotal junction or the proximal penile urethra. Straddle injuries compress the urethra against the symphysis pubis with possible rupture, therefore it is important to perform urethrography before attempting catheterization. A suprapubic catheter is the preferred option in this situation.
- Inflammation: usually occurs in the anterior urethra, often from gonorrhoea, tuberculosis or non-specific urethritis.
- Neoplasia: develop as a result of malignant infiltration, but is rare.

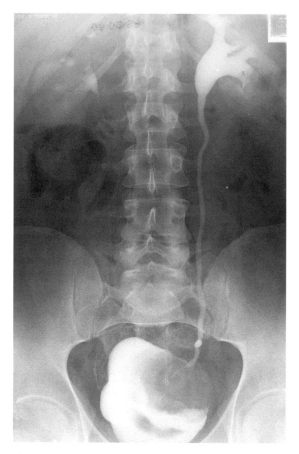

Fig. 6.36 IVU: carcinoma of the bladder seen as a filling defect in the left bladder; note renal obstruction.

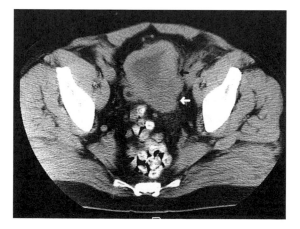

Fig. 6.37 CT shows left bladder wall thickening and extension of the carcinoma beyond the bladder wall (arrows).

BLADDER CARCINOMA

After prostatic carcinoma, the bladder is the commonest site of neoplastic involvement in the urinary tract. The tumour is usually a transitional cell carcinoma. Predisposing causes include:

- industrial exposure to aromatic amines;
- cigarette smoking;
- chronic infection with *Schistosoma haematobium* (squamous cell carcinoma);
- chronic inflammatory changes due to calculi (squamous cell carcinoma).

RADIOLOGICAL FEATURES

Cystoscopy is mandatory in any patient suffering from haematuria. IVU is also often performed to assess the upper urinary tract with respect to:

- degree of obstruction;
- state of the ureters;
- renal function;
- identifying other lesions as transitional cell carcinoma is often multifocal.

Demonstration of the bladder carcinoma is by either a filling defect in the contrast filled bladder or an irregular mucosal pattern on the postmicturition bladder films. If the intravenous urogram shows ureteric obstruction, it signifies muscular involvement near the ureteric orifice rather than obstruction by a neoplastic mass compressing the ureter. CT or MRI are useful in pre-operative assessment of intramural and extramural spread, local invasion, lymph-node enlargement, and liver or lung secondary deposits.

A chest X-ray should always be performed to exclude lung secondaries.

TREATMENT

Depends on the staging:

- Superficial tumours: Ta or T1 can be successfully resected endoscopically.
- Invasion of bladder muscle: T2, T3a, T3b may be treated by endoscopic resection, partial or total cystectomy with radiotherapy or chemotherapy.
- Invasion of surrounding organs: T4 into prostate, uterus etc. Need palliative radiotherapy or chemotherapy or palliative cystectomy with urinary diversion.

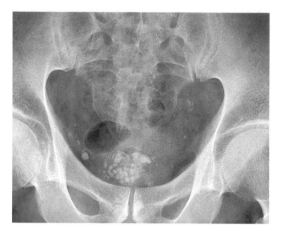

Fig. 6.38 Plain film shows prostatic calcification above the symphysis pubis.

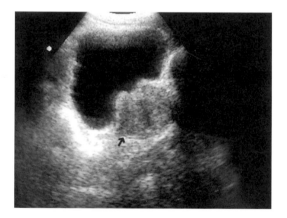

Fig. 6.39 Transabdominal ultrasound visualizing the prostate gland (arrow). Transrectal scanning is more accurate.

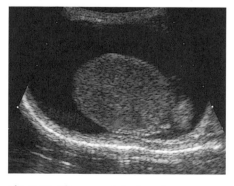

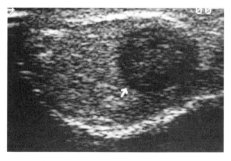

Fig. 6.41 Ultrsound: localized altered echo pattern in testicular tumour (arrow).

Fig. 6.40 Ultrasound: hydrocele, an occasional manifestation of testicular tumour.

PROSTATIC ENLARGEMENT

The usual cause of prostatic enlargement is benign hypertrophy but sometimes it may be due to carcinoma. Chronic retention secondary to outflow obstruction, as a result of prostatic enlargement, can lead to renal failure.

RADIOLOGICAL FEATURES

- *Plain films.* Prostatic calcification and calculi are common, seen as multiple fine-scattered densities projected above the symphysis pubis. Sclerotic secondary deposits from primary prostatic carcinoma may be visualized on a plain abdominal film.
- *Intravenous urography* may show a large filling defect at the bladder base, residual urine, the presence of obstructive changes and bladder wall thickening.
- *Transabdominal ultrasound.* Assesses upper urinary tract; it is more accurate than intravenous urography for residual urine.
- *Transrectal prostatic ultrasound.* The scan is performed after the introduction of the transducer into the rectum to assess the size and presence of localized masses. Differentiation between benign and neoplastic disease cannot be confidently made without a biopsy for histological analysis. Carcinomas are commonest in the periphery of the gland where they are seen as a focal nodule or diffuse infiltration.
- *CT/MRI.* Evaluates tumour spread beyond the prostatic capsule and tumour invasion into the bladder or rectum. MRI is proving the more precise technique.
- *Isotope bone scan.* May demonstrate secondary deposits.

TESTICULAR TUMOUR

Ultrasound is extremely effective in the evaluation of the normal testis and in recognizing a focal lesion; masses of only a few millimetres in diameter are accurately visualized. An abnormal echo lesion in the testis needs a biopsy for a definitive diagnosis.

- Seminoma: comprise the majority of testicular tumours and appear as homogeneous well-defined low echo mass lesions, sharply demarcated from normal testicular tissue.
- Teratoma: these have a mixed echo pattern and may be cystic or solid. The peak incidence of testicular tumours is between the ages of 25 and 35, with an increased risk in undescended testes. In the older age group, a testicular mass is more likely to be metastatic, rather than a primary tumour. Tumour staging requires a CT thorax, abdomen and pelvis.

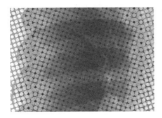

CHAPTER 7

Skeletal System and Fractures

SKELETAL SYSTEM: PROCEDURES

PLAIN FILMS

Plain films still remain the mainstay of radiological investigation of the skeletal system. Views should always be obtained in two projections.

ISOTOPES

Technetium-99m phosphonate compounds accumulate in bone several hours after intravenous injection of the isotope; principally used for:
- detection of osteomyelitis and other musculoskeletal soft-tissue inflammatory changes;
- metastatic bone lesions: changes are seen much earlier than plain films;
- staging tumours such as breast carcinoma or bronchial carcinoma;
- functional bone abnormality: Paget's disease.

Uptake of the isotope does occur, however, in many other conditions including osteoarthritis and inflammatory arthropathies.

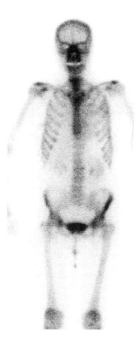

Fig. 7.1 Normal isotope bone scan.

ARTHROGRAPHY

In this procedure, contrast and air are injected into joints such as the knee, hip, elbow, shoulder, wrist and temporomandibular joints to diagnose loose bodies, ligamentous and cartilaginous abnormalities. The technique may be followed by computed tomography (CT arthrography). MRI is now the preferred modality in the majority of cases.

ULTRASOUND

Ultrasound is utilized for the evaluation of:

- neonatal hip for congenital dislocation;
- soft-tissue lesions, abscesses and masses;
- joint effusions.

CT

CT aids:

- assessment of bone tumours prior to surgery;
- evaluation of certain fractures, such as the acetabulum and subtalar joint;
- study of the spinal column.

MRI

Although bone is not adequately visualized from lack of a signal, marrow in cancellous bone produces very clear images. MRI assists the investigation of bone tumours, soft tissue masses, the spinal column and joints

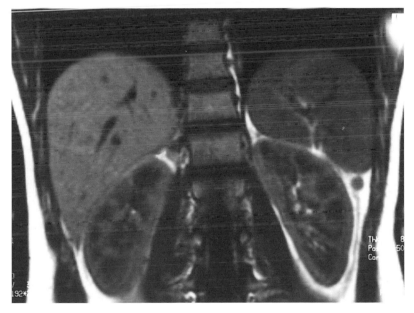

Fig. 7.2 MRI scan of the abdomen showing the thoraco-lumbar spine as well as the abdominal soft tissues, the liver, spleen, kidneys and psoas muscles.

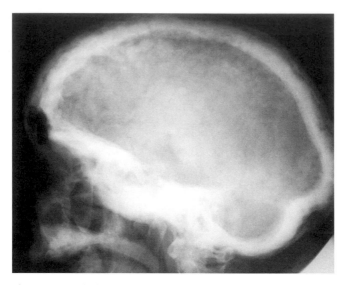

Fig. 7.3 Paget's disease: calvarial thickening producing a 'cotton wool' appearance.

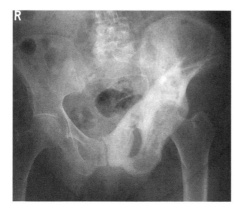

Fig. 7.4 Paget's disease of the left pelvis with marked bone expansion.

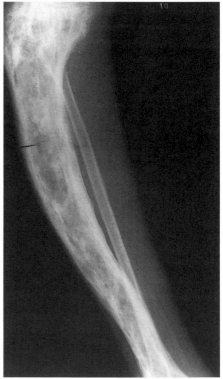

Fig. 7.5 Bowing of the tibia with pseudofracture in Paget's disease.

PAGET'S DISEASE

A common disorder of bone architecture, of unknown aetiology, which occurs with increasing frequency after middle age. It is characterized initially by bone resorption, followed by a reparative process in which increased bone deposition results in bone expansion and abnormal modelling.

PRESENTATION

Majority are asymptomatic and diagnosed as an incidental finding; bone pain; fractures; deformity of long bones and skull.

RADIOLOGICAL FEATURES

Any bone may be affected.
- Skull. Initially a large area of well defined bone loss may be seen (osteoporosis circumscripta); later, generalized sclerosis with diploic thickening produces a characteristic 'cotton wool' appearance. There may be an increase in the size of the head.
- Spine. Most commonly involves a single vertebra with sclerosis, altered trabecular pattern and enlargement of the vertebral body.
- Pelvis. Frequently affected with coarsened trabecular pattern, cortical thickening and enlargement of the pubis and ischium.
- Long bones. Widening of bone with deformities, bowing of the tibia and incomplete fractures because of bone softening.

COMPLICATIONS

- Pathological fractures: tend to be sharply transverse.
- Pseudofractures: incomplete fractures found on the convex surfaces of bowed bones.
- Secondary degenerative changes: the hip joint is most frequently involved.
- Malignant degeneration: in widespread Paget's disease there is an increased incidence of malignant bone tumours, especially osteogenic sarcoma.
- Neurological: nerve entrapment by bone expansion: deafness from VIIIth nerve involvement, encroachment of the spinal exit foramina, etc.
- Cardiovascular: increased shunting of blood in involved bone may cause high output failure, although this is rare.

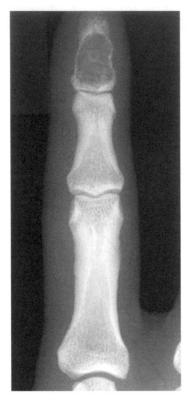

Fig. 7.6 Chondroma: a benign
cartilaginous tumour.

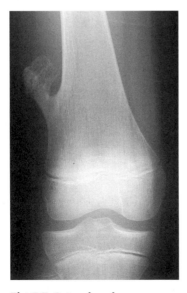

Fig. 7.7 Osteochondroma.

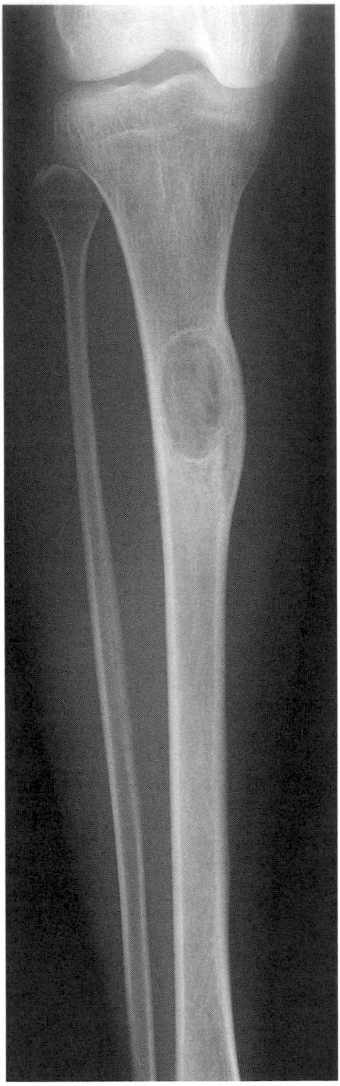

Fig. 7.8 Chondromyxoid
fibroma, a rare tumour but
demonstrates the features of
a benign tumour.

BENIGN BONE TUMOUR

Benign bone tumours are generally well defined and have a narrow zone of transition between normal and abnormal bone. They cause signs and symptoms by expansion and pressure on adjacent structures. If cystic, a pathological fracture may ensue.

CARTILAGE TUMOURS

Chondroma. A cartilaginous tumour, one of the most common benign tumours of bone, appears as a well-defined lytic lesion with small flecks of calcification. The hands and feet are most frequently affected, where expansion and thinning of the cortex may be a feature. Chondromas are often single but may be multiple in Ollier's disease.

Osteochondroma. Probably the commonest benign tumour, containing both bone and cartilage, often on a bony stalk with a bulbous broad distal end. The tumour is often found growing away from a joint, the most frequent site being the metaphyseal region of the lower femur and upper tibia. Hereditary multiple osteochondromas occur in diaphyseal aclasia, where a risk of malignant transformation to chondrosarcoma exists.

BONE FORMING TUMOURS

Osteoma. A benign tumour that contains only compact osseous tissue, most commonly found in the skull and sinuses. They are round, well defined and appear as a mass of amorphous dense bone with no cartilaginous component. Multiple osteomas are associated with colonic polyposis in Gardner's syndrome.

Osteoid osteoma. A small circular lucent area (nidus) under the cortex surrounded by thickened reactive bone and associated with periosteal reaction. Osteoid osteoma, a tumour of <1 cm in diameter, is usually a lesion of young adults and presents with local pain. It may be cored out under radiological control.

OTHER BENIGN LESIONS

Giant cell tumour. A benign tumour, with approximately half discovered in the vicinity of the knee joint. This is a lytic lesion of the epiphyseal region, with cortical thickening, expansion and the potential of turning into a malignant neoplasm.

Osteoblastoma; bone cyst; non-ossifying fibroma; aneurysmal bone cyst; chondromyxoid fibroma.

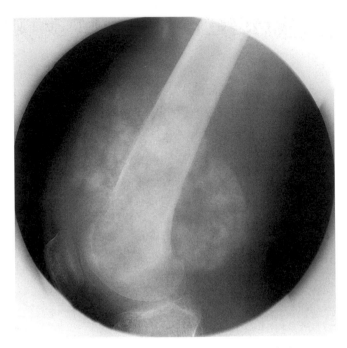

Fig. 7.9 Osteogenic sarcoma extending into the soft tissues.

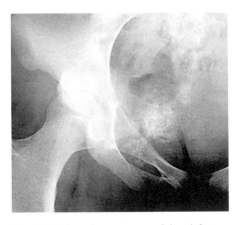

Fig. 7.10 Chondrosarcoma of the right pubic ramus.

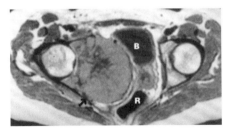

Fig. 7.12 MRI showing a large soft tissue component (arrow). B, bladder; R, rectum.

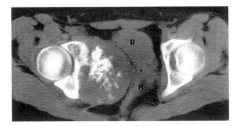

Fig. 7.11 CT scan demonstrating the tumour. B, bladder; R, rectum.

MALIGNANT BONE TUMOUR

Primary malignant bone tumours are uncommon: they are destructive, often associated with periosteal reactions, and have a wide zone of transition between normal and abnormal bone. The most common malignant bone tumour is a metastasis and it is often solitary.

RADIOLOGICAL FEATURES

Plain films may show an area of bone destruction.

CT and MRI are the best imaging modalities to evaluate tumours and determine bone and soft tissue involvement; definitive diagnosis is by a biopsy. Features that may be verified by CT/MRI are: tumour vascularity; infiltration of surrounding tissues; relationship to nerves and vessels.

MALIGNANT BONE TUMOURS

Osteosarcoma. The second most common primary malignant tumour of bone after multiple myeloma, the classical features being:

- irregular medullary destruction;
- periosteal reaction;
- cortical destruction;
- soft-tissue mass;
- new bone formation.

Osteosarcoma presents between the ages of 10 and 25. Approximately half appear around the knee joint, involving the metaphysis of the distal femur and proximal tibia. The tumour may be lytic in nature, or sclerotic with neoplastic new bone formation and periosteal reaction. It erodes from its origins in the medulla through the cortex, with a resulting soft-tissue mass. Metastases often spread to the lungs and may form bone.

Chondrosarcoma. A slow-growing malignant tumour, derived from cartilage cells, which may contain areas of calcification within the tumour.

- Central type: usually arise from a tubular bone, is lytic and situated in the region of the metaphysis.
- Peripheral type: probably originate from the periosteum or evolve from a previous benign osteochondroma.

Ewing's tumour. Presents between the ages of 5 and 15 years. A highly malignant tumour originating from bone marrow and associated with layered periosteal reactions (onion skin); the appearances may mimic an osteomyelitis.

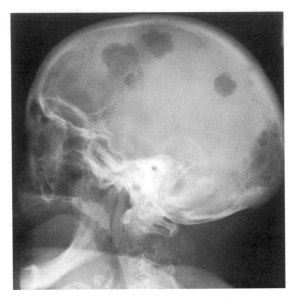

Fig. 7.13 Lytic deposits in the cranial vault.

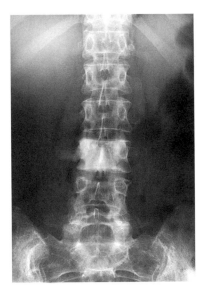

Fig. 7.14 Sclerotic deposit in a vertebral body.

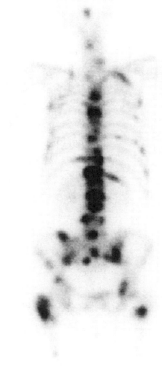

Fig. 7.15 (*right*) Isotope bone scan showing multiple bone deposits.

BONE METASTASES

Bone metastases are the most common malignant bone tumours. Metastases disseminate mainly to marrow-containing bones, therefore they are more commonly found in the axial skeleton. Generally, spread distal to the knee and elbow is less likely than the proximal skeleton. Any primary tumour may metastasize to bone, but the most frequent to do so are:
• Breast: high incidence of bone deposits, usually lytic in nature but may be sclerotic or mixed; the commonest cause of sclerotic deposits in females.
• Prostate: almost always sclerotic, lytic deposits being rare; the commonest cause of sclerotic deposits in a male.
• Lung: lytic deposits; peripheral deposits in the hands and feet are rare, but if present are likely to be from a bronchial carcinoma.
• Kidney, thyroid: lytic and can be highly vascular with bone expansion.
• Adrenal gland: predominantly lytic.

PRESENTATION

Bone pain; pathological fracture; soft-tissue swelling; staging or during follow-up of primary tumours.

RADIOLOGICAL FEATURES

Bone metastases tend to be either lytic or sclerotic. On plain films:
• Lytic deposits. Destruction of bone detail with poor definition of margins and associated pathological fractures are the principal features. Periosteal reactions are rare compared to primary malignant tumours.
• Sclerotic deposits. Show as an area of ill-defined increased density with subsequent loss of bone architecture. Vertebral secondaries may feature sclerotic pedicles. With multiple lesions, a diagnosis of metastases is almost certain. Isotope bone scanning is more sensitive than plain films (localized areas of increased uptake; hot spots).

In cases where the primary tumour is unknown, an image-guided biopsy of the bone lesion may reveal the site of the primary carcinoma.

DIFFERENTIAL DIAGNOSIS

• Paget's disease (sclerotic areas).
• Multiple myeloma (lytic areas).
• Primary malignant tumour.
• Infection or osteomyelitis.

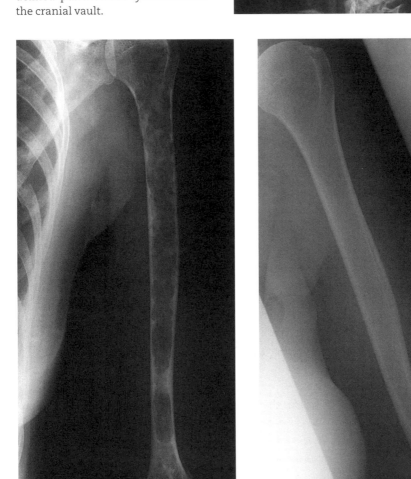

Fig. 7.16 Lateral skull in multiple myeloma showing widespread well-defined 'punched out' lytic lesions in the cranial vault.

Fig. 7.17 Myeloma deposits in the humerus producing lytic areas and 'endosteal scalloping': compare the appearances with a normal humerus.

MULTIPLE MYELOMA

Multiple myeloma is a primary malignant tumour of bone marrow, in which there is infiltration of the marrow-producing areas of the skeleton by a malignant proliferation of plasma cells. The skull, spine, pelvis, ribs, scapulae and the proximal axial skeleton are primarily involved with destruction of marrow and erosion of bony trabeculae; the distal skeleton is rarely involved. The disease may occur in a disseminated form, or as a localized solitary enlarging mass (plasmacytoma). Multiple myeloma is the most common primary malignant tumour of bone and tends to be confined to the skeletal system.

PRESENTATION

A male predominance, usually in the over-40 age group; weight loss; malaise; bone pain; backache; vertebral body collapse; pathological fracture; Bence–Jones proteinuria.

RADIOLOGICAL FEATURES

At time of presentation 80–90% have skeletal abnormalities. Plain films feature:

• Generalized osteoporosis with a prominence of the bony trabecular pattern, especially in the spine, resulting from marrow involvement with myeloma tissue. Loss of spinal bone density may be the only radiological sign in multiple myeloma. Pathological fractures are common.

• Compression fractures of the vertebral bodies, indistinguishable from those of senile osteoporosis.

• Scattered 'punched-out' lytic lesions with well-defined margins, those lying near the cortex produce internal scalloping.

• Bone expansion with extension through the cortex, producing soft-tissue masses.

COMPLICATIONS

• Pathological fractures that heal with abundant callus.
• Hypercalcaemia secondary to excessive bone destruction.
• Renal failure may result from a combination of amyloid deposition, hypercalcaemia and tubular precipitation of abnormal proteins.
• Increased incidence of infections such as pneumonia.
• Hyperuricaemia and secondary gout.

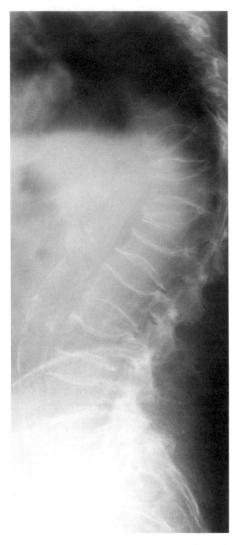

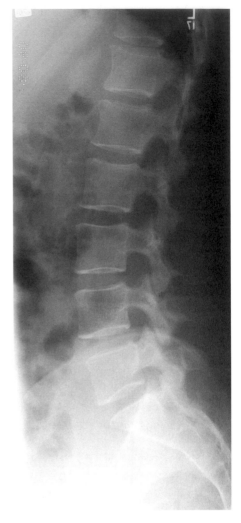

Fig. 7.19 Normal lumbar spine.

Fig. 7.18 Osteoporotic lower thoracic and
lumbar spine showing loss of bone
density with vertebral collapse.

OSTEOPOROSIS

Osteoporosis is a condition in which there is a reduction of bone mass.

PRESENTATION

- Asymptomatic.
- Bone pain.
- Skeletal fractures.
- Vertebral compression fractures.

RADIOLOGICAL INVESTIGATIONS

- Plain films.
- Bone densitometry either by CT, X-ray or isotope bone absorptiometry.

RADIOLOGICAL FEATURES

Detection of osteoporosis on plain films requires a reduction in bone mass of at least 25–30%. Osteoporosis results in a loss of bone density, a decrease in the number of trabeculae and coarse striations.

The condition manifests itself most prominently in the spine. The vertebral bodies appear lucent with thin cortical lines, often with a biconcave appearance ('cod fish' vertebrae), vertebral wedging and collapse; this subsequently leads to a kyphosis. Fractures of the peripheral skeleton, including femoral neck fractures, commonly occur even after minor trauma.

CAUSES OF LOCAL OSTEOPOROSIS

- Disuse of a particular part (tumours, fracture).
- Inflammatory conditions such as rheumatoid arthritis and osteomyelitis.
- Sudeck's atrophy (neural or muscle paralysis). Development of pain and osteoporosis often after slight trauma; it may have a neurovascular aetiology.

CAUSES OF GENERALIZED OSTEOPOROSIS

- Senile osteoporosis.
- Postmenopause.
- Steroid therapy.
- Immobility (prolonged bed rest).
- Endocrine: Cushing's disease.
- Multiple myeloma.
- Nutritional deficiency syndromes: scurvy, malnutrition, chronic liver disease, malabsorption syndromes.

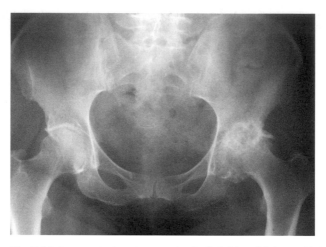

Fig. 7.20 Degenerative changes in the left hip with loss of joint space and osteophyte formation.

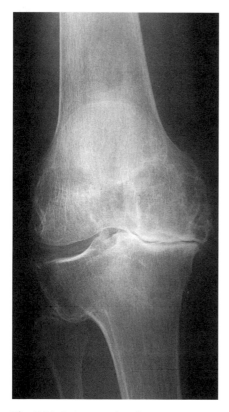

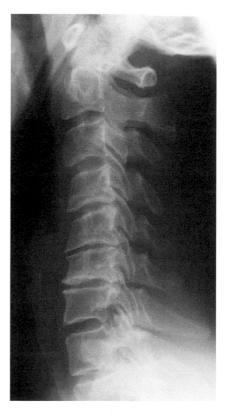

Fig. 7.21 Degenerative changes at the knee joint with loss of medial compartment joint space.

Fig. 7.22 Degenerative changes in the cervical spine with mid and lower cervical loss of disc space.

OSTEOARTHRITIS

Osteoarthritis is characterized by degeneration of articular cartilage and is part of the normal ageing process due to wear and tear of the articular surface. Secondary osteoarthritis results from previous trauma with malalignment of articular surfaces, joint infection and rheumatoid arthritis.

RADIOLOGICAL FEATURES

Any joint, particularly weight-bearing, may be affected. The hips, knees, shoulders, hands, wrists and spine are frequently involved. Features of osteoarthritis include:

• Osteophyte formation: osteophytes are spurs of compact bone which form at joint margins.
• Joint space narrowing: cartilage loss eventually leads to non-uniform joint space narrowing.
• Loose bodies: result from separation of cartilage and osteophytes.
• Subchondral cysts and sclerosis: increased bone density around joints with degenerative cyst formation.

COMMON SITES OF INVOLVEMENT

Knee. The most common joint involved, with femorotibial compartment loss of joint space. The medial compartment is the weight-bearing part under greatest stress, and so almost always shows the earliest narrowing. Severe changes may require total knee joint replacement.

Spine. Degenerative changes are present in nearly all elderly patients. Features include:

• narrowing of disc space;
• new bone formation (spurring) between adjacent vertebrae may cause nerve root impingement or spinal cord compression;
• sclerosis and osteophytes at intervertebral apophyseal joints.

Hips. Joint space narrowing is seen initially at the superior maximum weight-bearing aspect, with femoral and acetabular osteophytes. Other findings may include sclerosis and subchondral cyst formation. Severe changes often necessitate total hip joint replacement.

Hands. Typically affects:

• base of first metacarpal;
• proximal interphalangeal joints (Bouchard's nodes);
• distal interphalangeal joints (Heberden's nodes).

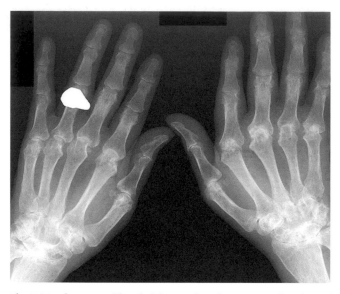

Fig. 7.23 Rheumatoid arthritis: erosive changes, predominantly at the metacarpo-phalangeal joints and wrists.

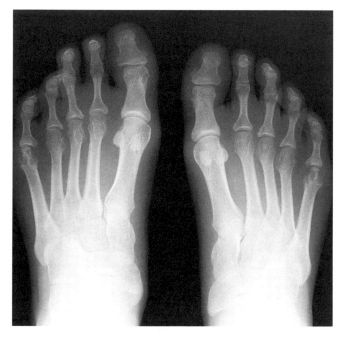

Fig. 7.24 Rheumatoid arthritis: symmetrical erosive changes at the heads of the fifth metatarsals.

RHEUMATOID ARTHRITIS

Rheumatoid arthritis is defined as a chronic polyarthritis due to inflammation, congestion and proliferation of synovium, leading to bone erosion with cartilage destruction.

RADIOLOGICAL FEATURES

Radiological changes lag behind clinical symptoms. Rheumatoid arthritis tends to have a symmetrical distribution, most commonly affecting the hands and feet. Any synovial joint may be involved, the most significant and frequent findings in rheumatoid arthritis being uniform narrowing of joint space, marginal erosions and periarticular osteoporosis.

The following features may be found:

• Joint swelling: from synovial membrane proliferation and joint effusions.

• Erosions: initially located in the periarticular area along the joint margins, where no protective layer exists. Erosions eventually spread across the articular surface.

• Osteoporosis: periarticular at first, but later generalized from disuse and hyperaemia.

• Joint-space narrowing: widening of joint spaces at the outset of disease, but eventually a significant narrowing from erosions and cartilage deformity. Obliteration and complete destruction of joint space eventually leads to ankylosis.

SPECIFIC SITES OF INVOLVEMENT

• Hands: the MCP and PIP joints are commonly affected, with distal interphalangeal joint involvement less marked. Abnormalities include soft-tissue swelling and subluxation at the MCP joints:

'Boutonnière' deformity: flexion deformity at proximal interphalangeal joint and extension at distal interphalangeal joint;

'Swan neck' deformity: hyperextension at proximal interphalangeal joint and flexion at distal interphalangeal joint.

• Feet: broadly similar changes to hands.

• Wrists: erosions with fusion of the carpal bones.

• Elbows: common site for soft-tissue rheumatoid nodules.

• Shoulders: erosion of humeral head and acromio-clavicular joints.

• Knees: uniform joint-space narrowing with osteoporosis. Baker's cyst is a complication, with rupture producing symptoms and signs similar to those of a deep-vein thrombosis.

• Cervical spine: subluxation, erosion and fusion. Subluxation is most common at the atlanto-axial joint.

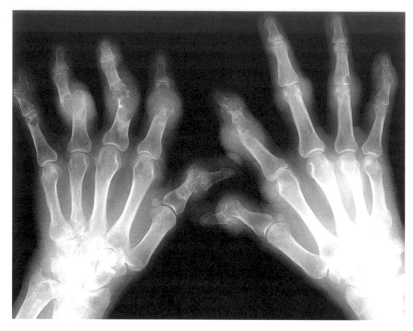

Fig. 7.25 Gout: soft tissue swelling with sharply defined erosions. Involvement is asymmetrical.

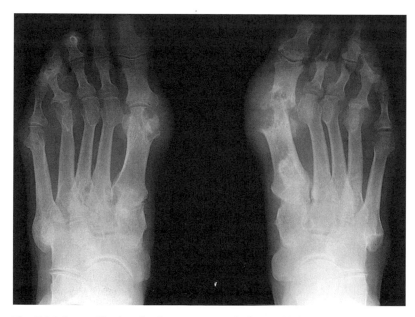

Fig. 7.26 Gout affecting the first metarso-phalangeal joints. Soft tissue swelling is present with large erosions.

GOUT

Gout is characterized by a raised plasma uric acid level with recurrent attacks of arthritis. It is due to an inborn error of metabolism and predominantly affects males.

PRESENTATION
- Hot swollen joint, usually the first metatarso-phalangeal (MTP) joint.
- Asymptomatic hyperuricaemia.

RADIOLOGICAL FEATURES
Radiological changes only occur many years after clinical symptoms. There exists a predilection for the first MTP joint, but ankles, knees, elbows and other joints may also be involved. Plain films may reveal:
- Joint effusions and swellings.
- Erosions: These tend to have a 'punched-out' appearance, lying separately from the articular surface. Bone density is preserved.
- Tophi: Composed of sodium urate and deposited in bone, soft tissues and around joints. Calcification in the tophi may be found, and intraosseous tophi may enlarge to produce erosions with joint destruction.

COMPLICATIONS
Renal calculi: non-opaque on plain films; renal failure.

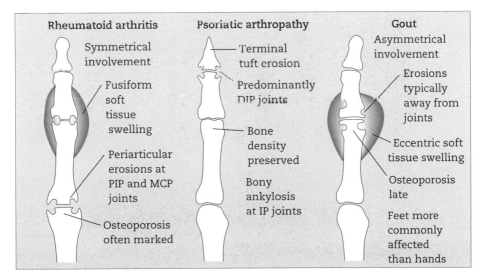

Fig. 7.27 Differential diagnosis of erosive arthropathy.

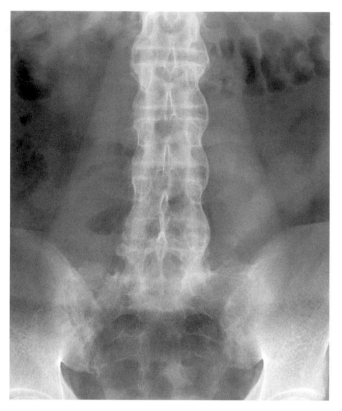

Fig. 7.28 Typical 'bamboo spine' with paraspinal ligament calcification. The right sacroiliac joint appears ill defined and the left fused.

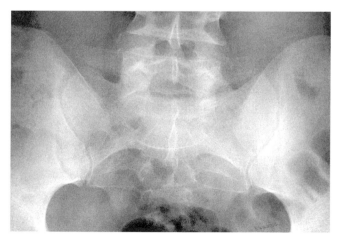

Fig. 7.29 Normal sacroiliac joints.

ANKYLOSING SPONDYLITIS

Ankylosing spondylitis, a progressive inflammatory disease, usually affects young adult males, often with a family history of the disease; 95% of patients carry the human leukocyte antigen (HLA-B27 antigen).

PRESENTATION

- Repeated attacks of backache and stiffness.
- Anorexia and weight loss.

RADIOLOGICAL FEATURES

On plain films the following features may be seen:

- *Sacroiliac joints.* The earliest changes begin in the sacroiliac joints with symmetrical blurring and poor definition of joint margins. Later, erosion and bony sclerosis lead to a tendency for complete sacroiliac joint fusion. Both joints are commonly affected; a unilateral sacroiliitis should raise the suspicion of a bacterial infection, commonly tuberculous. Sacroiliitis is usually evident on bone scanning before any radiographic change

- *Spinal changes.* The entire spine may be involved but changes usually commence in the lumbar region and progress upwards to involve the thoracic and cervical spine. The features most commonly noted are: squaring of the vertebral bodies due to new bone formation in the anterior vertebral bodies, and filling in of the normal anterior concavity by longitudinal ligamentous calcification; calcification of the lateral and anterior spinal ligaments to produce the classical 'bamboo spine'.

- *Peripheral joint involvement.* An erosive arthropathy may accompany ankylosing spondylitis, the hips being the commonest joints involved.

COMPLICATIONS/ASSOCIATIONS

- Upper-lobe lung fibrosis.
- Aortic incompetence: from an aortitis of the ascending aorta.
- Inflammatory bowel disease: a colitis resembling Crohn's disease or ulcerative colitis.
- Atlanto-axial subluxation.
- Fractures: spinal rigidity causes increased susceptibility to trauma.
- Ventilatory failure: due to restrictive chest movements and ankylosis of the costovertebral joints.
- Iritis.

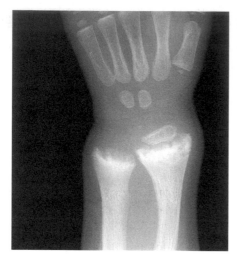

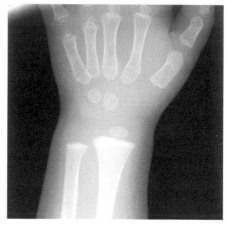

Fig. 7.31 Normal appearances in a child of similar age.

Fig. 7.30 Rickets in a 2-year-old child with widening and cupping of the distal radius.

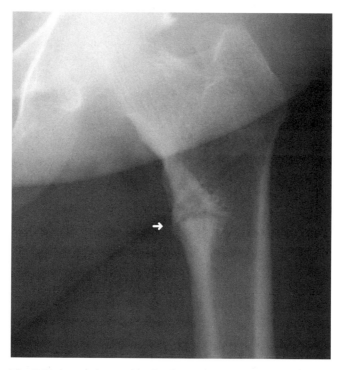

Fig. 7.32 'Looser's zone' in the femur (arrow).

RICKETS

Vitamin D deficiency in children can cause rickets. Deficiency may be nutritional, due to malabsorption, chronic renal disease or prolonged anticonvulsant therapy.

PRESENTATION

Failure to thrive; bone pain; bone deformities.

RADIOLOGICAL FEATURES

The principal pathological change is a lack of calcification of osteoid tissue in the growing epiphysis. The whole skeleton is affected, especially rapidly growing areas: wrists, knees and proximal humeri. Greenstick fractures are common.

The following features may be seen on plain films.

• Widening of the growth plate and epiphysis, with delayed appearance of epiphyses.

• Fraying and indistinct margins of the metaphysis producing a cupped appearance.

• Periosteal reactions, especially during the healing stage.

• Bowing and curvature of bones.

• Bulbous enlargement of the anterior ends of the ribs producing a 'rickety rosary'.

OSTEOMALACIA

Vitamin D deficiency in the mature skeleton can lead to osteomalacia, the adult counterpart of rickets.

PRESENTATION

Bone pain; muscular weakness; elevated serum alkaline phosphatase; pathological fractures.

RADIOLOGICAL FEATURES

• Generalized reduction in bone density.

• Looser's zones (pseudofractures) are narrow translucent bands, at the cortical margins, and are diagnostic of osteomalacia. They are seen most frequently in the ribs, scapulae, pubic rami and medial aspects of the proximal femora.

• Biconcave vertebrae ('cod fish' vertebrae).

• Bone softening leading to triradiate pelvis.

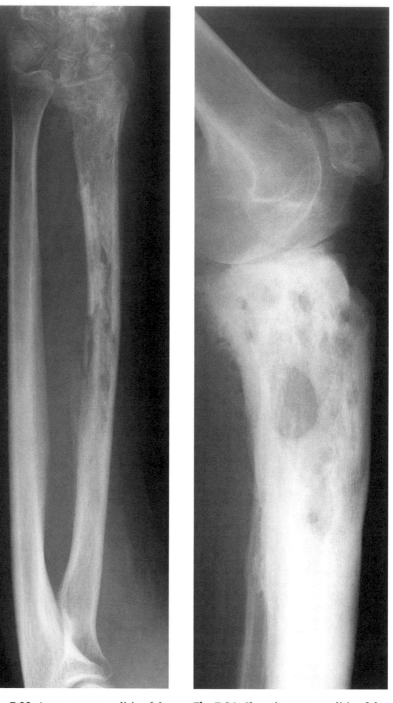

Fig. 7.33 Acute osteomyelitis of the radius with patchy bone destruction.

Fig. 7.34 Chronic osteomyelitis of the tibia with extensive sclerosis.

OSTEOMYELITIS

Osteomyelitis is an infection of bone, *Staphylococcus aureus* being responsible for the majority of cases; other causes include tuberculosis and *Salmonella* infection in sickle cell disease. The inflammatory process can be either acute or chronic, the latter leading to bone necrosis and pus formation, which sometimes discharges through to the skin to form a sinus communication with bone. Necrotic bone may separate from living tissue to produce a sequestrum. Sources of infection may be:

- haematogenous: usually in children;
- direct traumatic implantation, e.g. compound fracture or surgery;
- extension from adjacent soft tissues, e.g. a foot ulcer in diabetes.

PRESENTATION

- Pain.
- Pyrexia.

RADIOLOGICAL FEATURES

- *Plain films*: may be normal for up to 10 days but the earliest sign is soft-tissue swelling. Infected bone initially loses detail and becomes ill-defined with periosteal reaction and eventually bone destruction.
- *Isotope bone scanning*: uses technetium, gallium or labelled white cells. All indicate increased activity but are non-specific as conditions such as Paget's disease or neoplasia may also show increased uptake. The findings have to be interpreted in the clinical setting.
- *CT*: detects associated soft-tissue mass and sequestra. Their presence may need surgical removal.
- *MRI*: a sensitive technique in detecting infection.

Chronic osteomyelitis

Organisms responsible for the infection persist in dead bone, and exacerbations may ensue periodically. The bone appears thickened and sclerotic with a central radiolucent destructive area, often with a chronic draining sinus. An abscess with a sclerotic margin, sometimes containing a sequestrum, may follow (Brodie's abscess).

COMPLICATIONS

- Soft-tissue abscess.
- Fistulae.
- Premature fusion of epiphyses.
- Deformity.
- Pyogenic arthritis leading to bony ankylosis (e.g. hip fusion).

FRACTURES

Plain films are the principal method of initial evaluation of a patient with suspected skeletal trauma. Any bone may fracture but some are particularly susceptible. Typical signs and features of a fracture are:

• Fracture line: the fracture line may traverse the whole diameter of the bone or minor fractures may cause a break in the continuity of the normal cortical outline.

• Soft tissue swelling: usually accompanies a fracture.

• Cortical irregularity: a slight bulge or step in the cortex.

TYPES OF FRACTURES

• Greenstick: in children bone tends to be flexible, so a fracture may occur with buckling or bending of bone or a break only on one side of the cortex.

• Comminuted: a fracture with multiple fragments.

• Avulsion: a fragment of bone becomes detached from the site of a ligamentous or tendon insertion.

• Pathological: a fracture through diseased bone, often after trivial trauma, e.g. Paget's disease, osteoporosis or tumour.

• Stress or fatigue fracture: results from chronic repetitive minor trauma. Susceptible areas include the second and third metatarsals (march fracture), proximal tibial shaft and the base of the fifth metatarsal.

• Impacted fracture: the fragments are compressed into each other.

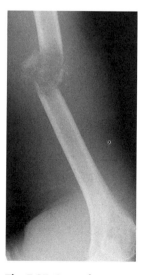 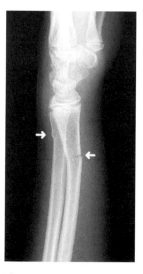

Fig. 7.35 Secondary deposit in the humerus; pathological fracture.

Fig. 7.36 Greenstick fractures of the distal forearm (arrows).

Skull fractures

- Linear: sharply defined linear lucency.
- Depressed: bony fragment thrust inwards with inner table depressed by greater than thickness of the cranial vault.

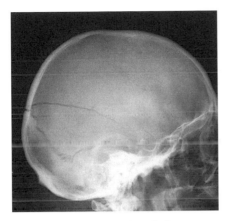

Fig. 7.37 Linear cranial vault fractures.

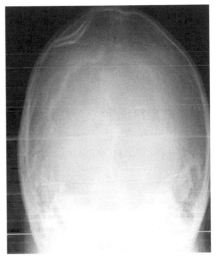

Fig. 7.38 Depressed skull fracture.

Cervical spine

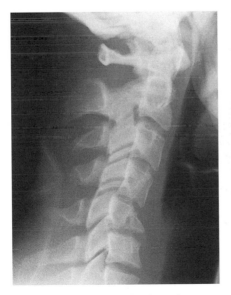

Fig. 7.39 Cervical vertebral crush fracture of C5 following trauma.

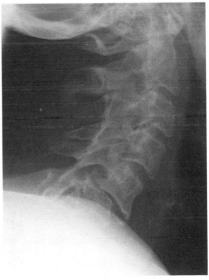

Fig. 7.40 Cervical spine subluxation at C5/C6.

Shoulder dislocation

Shoulder dislocation commonly results from an athletic injury or fall. Dislocation almost always occurs anteriorly with the humeral head lying in front of, and below, the glenoid cavity; posterior dislocation is rare. Avulsion of the glenoid labrum or avulsion of the greater tuberosity may be associated with the dislocation. Complications include damage to the radial and axillary nerves or rotator cuff muscles.

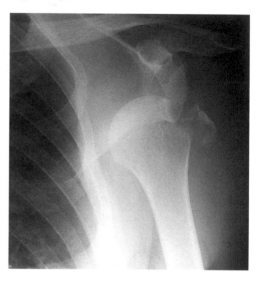

Fig. 7.41 Anterior dislocation with a fracture of the greater tuberosity.

Humeral neck fracture

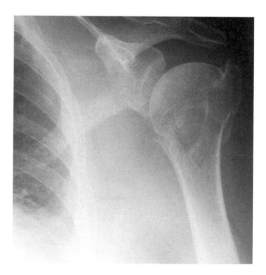

Fig. 7.42 Humeral neck fracture.

Supracondylar fracture

Usually occur in children; brachial artery injury is a recognized complication.

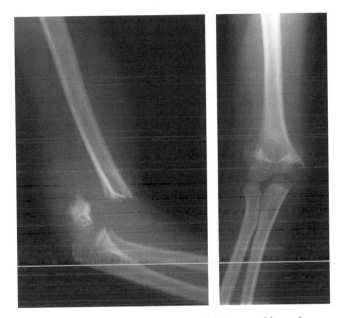

Fig. 7.43 Severe supracondylar fracture in a young child, AP and lateral projections.

Elbow fractures

These can be classified as: intercondylar T and Y fractures; lateral and medial condylar fracture; radial head fracture; olecranon fracture; and elbow dislocation.

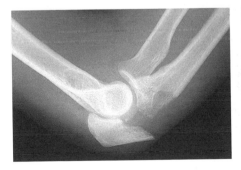
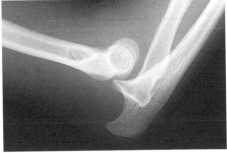

Fig. 7.44 Olecranon fracture.   **Fig. 7.45** Dislocation at the elbow.

Colles' fracture

May follow a fall on the outstretched hand, resulting in a fracture of the lower end of the radius with posterior displacement of the distal fragment.

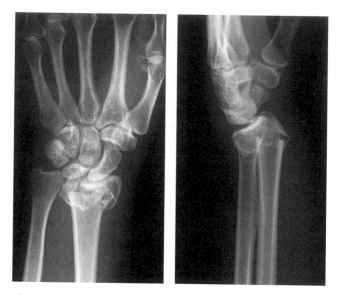

Fig. 7.46 Colles' fracture.

Scaphoid fracture

The fracture is often difficult to identify and if there is clinical suspicion, a further X-ray after 10 days is required, when it may be more easily visualized. Complications include non-union and avascular necrosis of the proximal fragment.

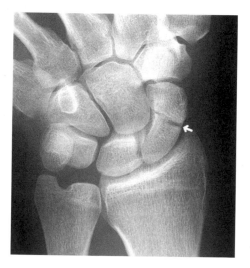

Fig. 7.47 Scaphoid fracture (arrow).

Hip fracture

Fractures can be classified into femoral neck, trochanteric and sub-trochanteric types.

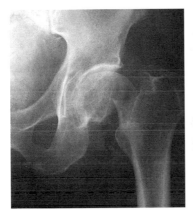

Fig. 7.48 Femoral neck fracture.

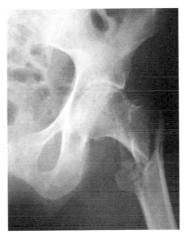

Fig. 7.49 Intertrochanteric fracture.

Ankle fracture

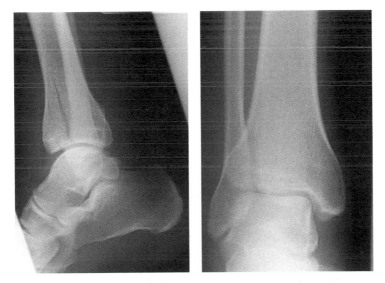

Fig. 7.50 Fracture of the medial malleolus, seen only on the lateral view showing the importance of two projections.

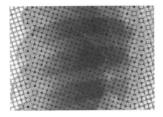

CHAPTER 8

Paediatrics

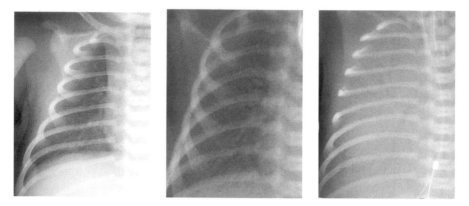

Fig. 8.1 Normal neonatal chest progressing to mild and then severe hyaline membrane disease.

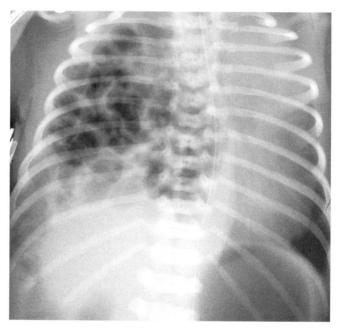

Fig. 8.2 Congenital diaphragmatic hernia: multiple bowel loops in the right thorax.

HYALINE MEMBRANE DISEASE

This is the most common cause of respiratory distress in premature births due to deficiency of pulmonary surfactant preventing alveolar distension. Transudation into the alveolar space and a lining of debris and dead cells (hyaline membrane) impairs gaseous exchange.

RADIOLOGICAL FEATURES

A chest X-ray may illustrate the following:
- typical ground glass or a fine granular appearance to the lungs;
- air bronchogram;
- low volume lungs.

COMPLICATIONS

Pneumothorax; pneumomediastinum and pulmonary interstitial emphysema from overdistended alveoli leaking air.

TREATMENT

- Positive pressure ventilation to maintain patency of terminal alveoli and preserve oxygenation.
- Surfactant given via the endotracheal tube in ventilated babies.

CONGENITAL DIAPHRAGMATIC HERNIA

A congenital defect in the diaphragm, more common on the left, allows bowel protrusion into the thoracic cavity and usually results in respiratory distress. Herniation may occur at three sites though those causing neonatal respiratory distress are usually of the Bochdalek type.
- Foramen of Bochdalek: posterior diaphragm.
- Foramen of Morgagni: anterior diaphragm.
- Oesophageal hiatus

RADIOLOGICAL FEATURES

Antenatal ultrasound examination often detects the herniation. A chest X-ray illustrates either cyst-like changes or the typical appearance of multiple bowel loops in the thorax. Mediastinal shift is away from the affected side. Abdominal films may show absence or paucity of bowel loops.

TREATMENT

Surgical repair of the diaphragm, but pulmonary hypoplasia and pulmonary hypertension cause a significant mortality.

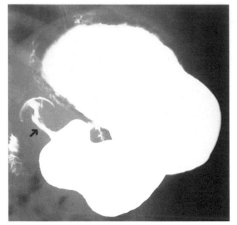

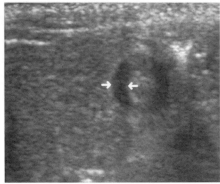

Fig. 8.4 Transverse ultrasound section of the pylorus with muscle thickening (arrows).

Fig. 8.3 Pyloric stenosis: contrast examination of the stomach showing a narrowed elongated pyloric canal (arrow).

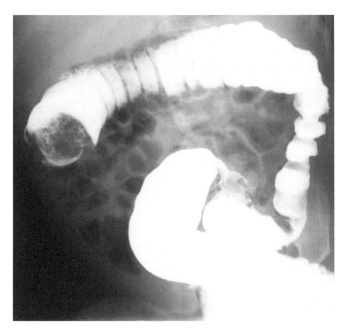

Fig. 8.5 Barium enema demonstrates obstruction in the mid-transverse colon by an intussusception.

PYLORIC STENOSIS

Pyloric stenosis is characterized by smooth-muscle hypertrophy of the pyloric muscle. It usually presents between 3 and 6 weeks after birth, with a marked male:female preponderance in its incidence (4:1). Pyloric stenosis is a clinical diagnosis, the pyloric mass often being palpable, but in doubtful cases an ultrasound or a water-soluble contrast meal are often diagnostic. Treatment is by a myotomy of the pyloric muscle: Ramstedt's operation.

PRESENTATION
- Vomiting (often projectile and not bile stained).
- Dehydration.
- Hypochloraemic alkalosis.
- Failure to thrive.

RADIOLOGICAL FEATURES
Ultrasound demonstrates the pyloric canal with the surrounding thickened muscle. *Water-soluble contrast examination* of the stomach shows delayed gastric emptying with an elongation and narrowing of the pyloric canal.

INTUSSUSCEPTION

An intussusception results from telescoping or invagination of one segment of bowel into another, producing obstructive changes. It is most common in the ileocaecal area and may be clinically palpable. Bowel infarction will ensue if left untreated.

PRESENTATION
Occur most frequently in children up to 2-years of age: drowsiness; colicky abdominal pain; vomiting; blood per rectum.

RADIOLOGICAL FEATURES
- Plain films may reveal signs of small bowel obstruction and a soft tissue mass caused by the head of the intussusception.
- Ultrasound, a non-invasive test, may identify the abdominal mass.
- Barium enema, however, is necessary for a definitive diagnosis. The diagnostic feature is complete obstruction to the flow of barium, with a crecentic filling defect at the site of obstruction.

TREATMENT
A high success rate follows radiologically controlled hydrostatic reduction using barium or air. If this fails, surgical reduction is necessary.

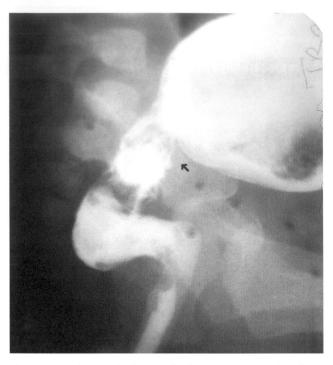

Fig. 8.6 Hirschprung's disease: barium enema showing the transition zone in the upper rectum (arrow).

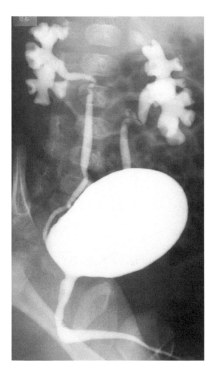

Fig. 8.7 Gross bilateral vesico-ureteric reflux as the child is micturating.

HIRSCHSPRUNG'S DISEASE

In Hirschsprung's disease, an aganglionic segment of colon with a deficiency or absence of the myenteric plexus, results in a non-distensible section, the proximal large bowel dilating and eventually resulting in a 'megacolon'. Rarely, agangliosis may affect the whole of the large bowel. Diagnosis is by a rectal biopsy. Complications include necrotizing enterocolitis and caecal perforation secondary to distension and ischaemia.

PRESENTATION

- Failure to pass meconium within 24 hours, with signs of intestinal obstruction: abdominal distension and vomiting.
- Constipation dating from birth; presentation may be in infancy or in later life.

RADIOLOGICAL FEATURES

Plain abdominal films reveal a grossly dilated redundant colon loaded with faecal residue. On barium enema examination, the involved segment is usually of a normal calibre (transition zone) but appears narrow, due to the distended colon above. Retention of barium for up to 48 hours after the examination is a typical feature.

VESICO-URETERIC REFLUX

The normal vesico-ureteric junction does not allow backward flow of urine from the bladder into the ureter. With reflux, the junction is incompetent and urine flows retrogradely up the ureters, especially during micturition. Reflux tends to resolve spontaneously during childhood, but is important to recognize because when associated with infection, chronic renal scarring may result. Urinary-tract infection needs to be controlled in the presence of reflux, in order to prevent retardation of renal growth.

RADIOLOGICAL FEATURES

With severe reflux, isotope scanning, ultrasound and micturating cystourethrography may reveal the following:
- upper urinary tract dilatation;
- renal atrophy;
- renal scarring with loss of cortical tissue, especially at the upper pole.

TREATMENT

- Low-dose antibiotics to maintain a sterile urine.
- Surgical re-implantation of the ureters in difficult cases.

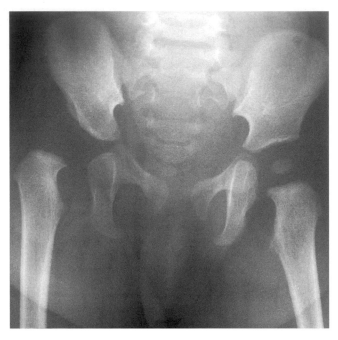

Fig. 8.8 Dislocation of the right hip. There is a delay in the appearance of the ossification centre of the femoral head.

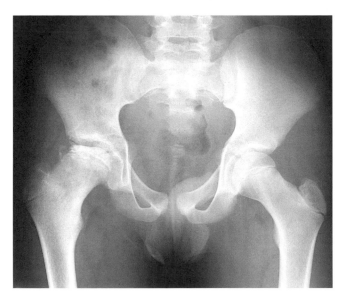

Fig. 8.9 Perthes' disease: flattening and increased density of the right femoral head.

CONGENITAL DISLOCATION OF HIPS

Congenital dislocation of the hips more commonly affects females. Numerous factors may play a part in the aetiology of this condition, including genetic causes and breech presentation.

RADIOLOGICAL INVESTIGATIONS

Ultrasound; plain films of the pelvis.

RADIOLOGICAL FEATURES

At birth, films of the pelvis are of little help as the femoral head is not ossified. Ultrasound may demonstrate a shallow acetabulum and determine its slope; it visualizes the position of the femoral head, and any subluxation or dislocation. Ultrasound can also monitor treatment ensuring that the hip remains stable.

Plain films are more useful at a later stage, when there is ossification of the femoral head nucleus. Features to note are a delayed appearance of the ossific nucleus, a shallow acetabulum and displacement of the femoral head upwards and laterally from its normal position.

PERTHES' DISEASE

Perthes' disease is an osteonecrosis (osteochondritis) of the epiphysis of the femoral head likely to be due to a deficient blood supply. It is five times commoner in males, with a peak incidence at 4–8 years and 10% of cases may be bilateral. Hip pain and limp are the main presenting features. Trauma and previous surgical reduction of a congenital dislocation of the hip are aetiological factors.

RADIOLOGICAL FEATURES

The following appearances may be seen in the femoral head on plain films:
* reduction in size;
* increased density;
* fragmentation and condensation;
* persistent deformity after healing with associated thickening of the femoral neck.

MRI can detect avascular necrosis earlier than plain films and may be useful to assess progress and treatment.

COMPLICATIONS

Degenerative disease in adulthood.

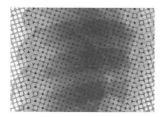

CHAPTER 9

Obstetrics and Gynaecology

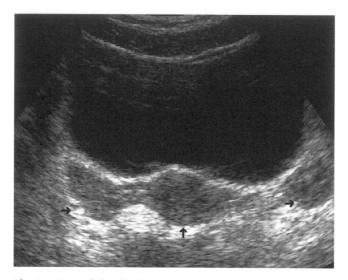

Fig. 9.1 Transabdominal scan demonstrating the midline uterus (↑) and ovaries (→) on either side.

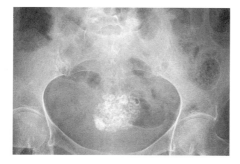

Fig. 9.2 Calcification in a fibroid.

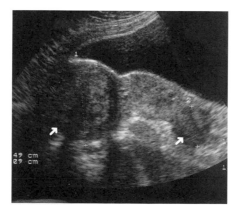

Fig. 9.3 Ultrasound examination demonstrating two large fibroids (arrows) in the uterus.

NORMAL UTERUS AND OVARIES

The uterus and ovaries are well visualized by a pelvic ultrasound scan. A more precise and detailed examination is obtained using a transvaginal probe.

• Uterus: ultrasound assesses size, outline, position and myometrial abnormalities such as leiomyomas and congenital uterine anomalies.

• Endometrium: this is seen as an echogenic linear area, the appearances varying through the menstrual cycle. It is poorly visualized in post-menopausal women due to atrophic changes and carcinoma may be suspected when there is abnormal thickening or configuration.

• Endometrial cavity: ultrasound accurately delineates retained products of conception and may visualize polyps.

• Fallopian tubes: generally not adequately seen, unless there is a hydrosalpinx.

• Ovaries: appear as oval structures lateral to the uterus, being small and atrophic in postmenopausal women. Follicular development can be monitored using ultrasound.

• Adnexa, cul-de-sac: detection of masses and free fluid.

UTERINE FIBROIDS (LEIOMYOMA)

Fibroids are common tumours, resulting from benign overgrowth of smooth muscle and connective tissue.

RADIOLOGICAL FEATURES

The following may be noted on ultrasound.

• Calcification: also shown on plain films and computed tomography (CT).

• Enlarged uterus, with a distorted outline.

• Lobular or round masses of variable echogenicity being either myometrial, pedunculated or subendometrial.

Magnetic resonance imaging (MRI) is more sensitive at detecting fibroids (90%) than ultrasound (60%).

COMPLICATIONS

• Infertility.

• Dystocia.

• Malignant sarcomatous degeneration (rare).

• Cystic degeneration.

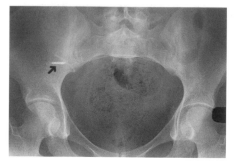

Fig. 9.4 Perforation with IUCD seen lying over the right iliac bone (arrow).

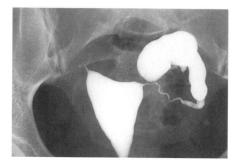

Fig. 9.5 Hysterosalpingography: occlusion of the right fallopian tube and a left hydrosalpinx.

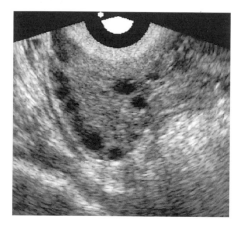

Fig. 9.6 Polycystic ovary: transvaginal scan demonstrating an enlarged ovary with multiple small cysts.

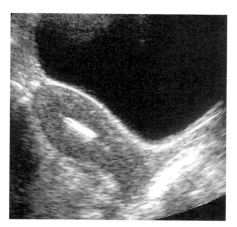

Fig. 9.7 Ultrasound: IUCD in the endometrial cavity.

INTRAUTERINE CONTRACEPTIVE DEVICE

Ultrasound is a valuable aid in assessing the position of an intrauterine contraceptive device (IUCD), identified lying in the endometrial cavity as a linear echogenic structure. The commonest cause of non-visualization is, however, expulsion of the device. If not seen on ultrasound, a plain abdominal film is recommended, as the IUCD may have perforated through the myometrium and be lying free in the abdominal cavity. Perforation is usually silent without symptoms and the IUCD can be removed by laparoscopy.

FALLOPIAN-TUBE OCCLUSION

Causes of occluded fallopian tubes include previous infection, peritonitis (especially from appendicitis) or tubal surgery. Radiological confirmation can be obtained by hysterosalpingography, the injection of contrast into the uterine cavity to assess the uterus and patency of fallopian tubes. Usually there is rapid filling of the fallopian tubes with free spillage of contrast into the peritoneal cavity, confirming tubal patency.

POLYCYSTIC OVARIES

Polycystic ovaries are associated with chronic anovulation due to disturbances of leuteinizing hormone (LH) and follicle stimulating hormone (FSH).

The classical clinical features that suggest polycystic ovary syndrome are obesity, hirsuitism, infertility and oligomenorrhoea (Stein–Leventhal syndrome). However, many women have biochemical abnormalities without these features, and present with menstrual irregularity.

Ultrasound may show marked ovarian enlargement, although they may be of a normal size. Multiple small immature follicles are noted, often lying in the subcapsular position.

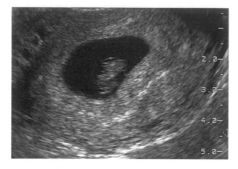

Fig. 9.8 Gestation at 6 weeks.

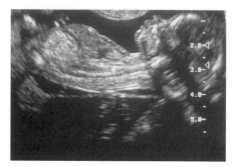

Fig. 9.9 Gestation at 16 weeks.

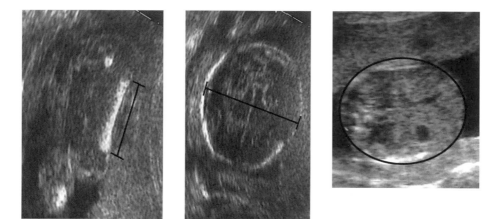

Fig. 9.10 Fetal measurements on ultrasound: femur length, biparietal diameter and abdominal circumference.

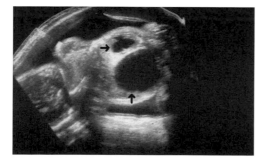

Fig. 9.11 Ultrasound demonstrating a distended fetal bladder (↑) with a hydronephrotic kidney (→).

GESTATION: 6 WEEKS

Ultrasound can be performed to confirm and date pregnancy or to detect complications such as an ectopic pregnancy or threatened abortion. The earliest detection of the sac is at 5–6 weeks on a pelvic ultrasound scan, seen as a ring-shaped echo-free area in the uterine cavity. Gestation age can be estimated by sac volume and the fetal crown–rump length; fetal cardiac pulsation is visible at approximately 7 weeks.

Transvaginal scanning produces a more detailed evaluation and both the gestation sac and cardiac pulsation are recognized earlier than with a transabdominal scan.

GESTATION: 16 WEEKS

Ultrasound is often used at this time to assess gestation age, fetal viability and fetal abnormalities. The placenta can be evaluated for its location and any accompanying abnormalities.

Fetal parameters utilized for gestation age are:
- biparietal diameter;
- head circumference;
- abdominal circumference;
- femur length.

FETAL ANOMALY

A vast number of fetal abnormalities can be detected by ultrasound some of which include:
- central nervous system: anencephaly, spina bifida, meningocele, encephalocele and hydrocephalus;
- chest: cardiac anomalies and pulmonary hypoplasia;
- gastrointestinal tract: duodenal atresia;
- renal tract: hydronephrosis, polycystic disease;
- skeletal: dwarfism.

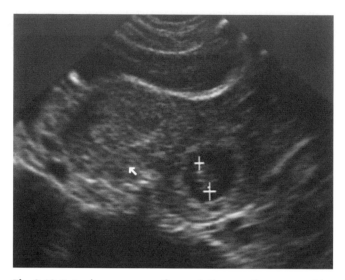

Fig. 9.12 Ectopic pregnancy: the gestation sac (between ++) is seen outside the uterus (arrow).

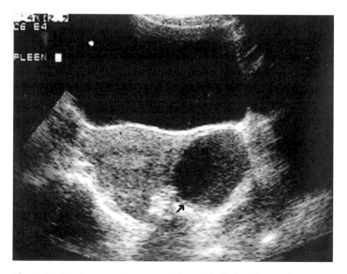

Fig. 9.13 Benign ovarian cyst: thin walled simple cystic structure (arrow) seen adjacent to the uterus.

ECTOPIC GESTATION

Ectopic pregnancy arises from failure of a fertilized ovum to reach the uterine cavity with subsequent implantation in the fallopian tube. Rarely, implantation may occur in the ovary or peritoneal cavity. An increased risk of ectopic pregnancy exists with pelvic inflammatory disease, use of an IUCD and a previous history of tubal surgery or ectopic gestation.

RADIOLOGICAL FEATURES

A normal ultrasound examination does not exclude an ectopic pregnancy, evaluation being more precise using transvaginal scanning. Some of the features below may be present:

- absence of gestation sac in uterine cavity (with positive pregnancy test);
- visualization of gestation sac or fetus outside the uterine cavity;
- endometrial thickening;
- free pelvic fluid;
- adnexal mass.

The tubal pregnancy often ceases at 6–10 weeks either by tubal rupture or tubal abortion.

BENIGN OVARIAN CYST

Ovarian cysts are common and they can attain sizes that can occupy most of the abdominal cavity.

RADIOLOGICAL FEATURES

On ultrasound the typical appearances indicating a benign lesion are: thin walls; free of internal echoes; lack of internal septations.

Simple cysts ≤6 cm should have a follow-up ultrasound. A large cyst may show on a plain abdominal film as a soft-tissue mass arising out of the pelvis. Complex cysts may be haemorrhagic or endometrioma.

CT and MRI are both accurate imaging modalities when ultrasound is equivocal or when malignancy is suspected.

TYPES OF BENIGN CYSTS

- Follicular cysts. These are unruptured graffian follicles. They resolve spontaneously and generally do not attain a size ≥6 cm. Serial scans confirm resolution of these cysts.
- Corpus luteum cysts. The corpus luteum normally degenerates after ovulation, but may persist, sometimes with internal haemorrhage.
- Mucinous cystadenoma and serous cystadenoma are benign cysts with a malignant potential, a far more frequent occurrence in the latter.

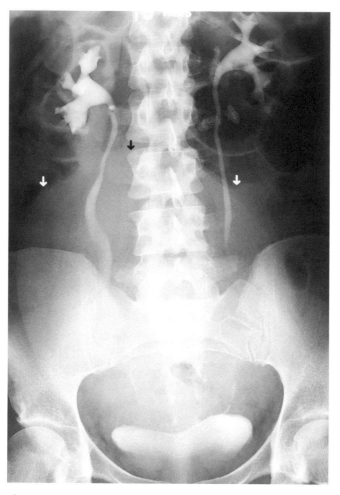

Fig. 9.14 Ovarian carcinoma: large mass seen arising out of the pelvis (arrows) and causing moderate ureteric obstruction.

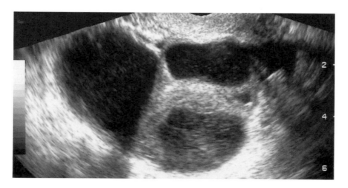

Fig. 9.15 Cystadenocarcinoma: ultrasound demonstrating a large cystic lesion with several internal septations.

OVARIAN CARCINOMA

Ovarian carcinoma is the commonest cause of death from female genital-tract cancer.

PRESENTATION

- Asymptomatic discovery on routine examination.
- Weight loss and anorexia.
- Abnormal vaginal bleeding.
- Pelvic abdominal mass or distension.

RADIOLOGICAL INVESTIGATIONS

- Plain abdomen; chest X ray.
- Ultrasound.
- Intravenous urography (IVU).
- MRI/CT for staging.

RADIOLOGICAL FEATURES

- *Ultrasound* is the most appropriate initial investigation and the diagnosis can be frequently made by this technique. Malignancy may be suspected in a pelvic mass if the following features are present: thick irregular septations with nodules; thick wall with irregularity of the inner wall; mixed solid and cystic components; local invasion; ascites (although this may also be seen in benign lesions); liver metastases.
- *IVU* is performed if there is suspicion of ureteric involvement.
- *MRI/CT* are accurate in staging the tumour prior to resection.

COMPLICATIONS

- Torsion: twisting on its pedicle interrupts the blood supply, initially venous then arterial. Results in severe pain when this complication arises.
- Infection.
- Rupture: pain and vomiting.
- Haemorrhage into cyst.

MALIGNANT OVARIAN TUMOURS

- Metastases: Krukenberg secondaries from mucus-secreting stomach or colon carcinoma.
- Malignant cystadenocarcinoma.
- Granulosa cell, theca cell, androblastoma, disgerminoma, teratoma.

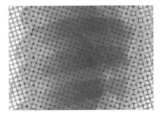

CHAPTER 10

Neuroradiology

NEURORADIOLOGY: INVESTIGATIONS

PLAIN FILMS

The need for plain skull films in diagnosis has virtually disappeared. They may show:

• calcification: glioma, meningioma, anteriovenous malformation, post-infective foci:

   pituitary fossa enlargement;

   lytic bone deposits;

   fractures;

• Plain spine films are initially utilized in the evaluation of trauma, they are generally not helpful in back pain.

ULTRASOUND

The neonatal brain can be imaged through the open anterior fontanelle for intraventricular haemorrhage, hydrocephalus or other suspected intracranial pathology. Carotid Doppler studies are used for the diagnosis of carotid stenosis.

COMPUTED TOMOGRAPHY (CT)

A typical brain study is carried out using 5–10 mm sections with approximately 14 slices per examination. High-definition 1 or 2 mm sections are taken where detail is needed, for example the pituitary fossa, internal auditory meati or orbits. In spinal CT demonstration of bony canal stenosis and disc prolapse are the two principal indications.

MAGNETIC RESONANCE IMAGING (MRI)

MRI scans demonstrate the brain using a multiplanar facility in axial, coronal and sagittal planes with excellent views of the posterior fossa, as there are no bone artefacts. It is a particularly sensitive investigation in the detection of tumours such as pituitary adenomas and acoustic neuroma. MRI is superior to CT in many situations including:

• lesions of pituitary fossa;
• spinal cord;
• visualization of demyelinating plaques in multiple sclerosis;
• differentiation of grey and white matter;
• identification of the lesional causes of epilepsy.

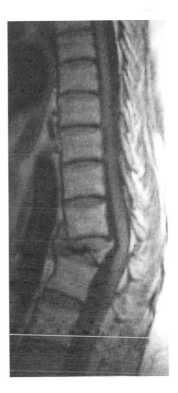

Fig. 10.1 MRI: vertebral collapse of T12 causing early spinal cord compression.

ARTERIOGRAPHY

Arteries of the cerebral circulation may be visualized by:

• digital subtraction angiography (DSA) with contrast injection in the superior vena cava or aortic arch;

• selective injection of contrast into the carotid and vertebral arteries;

• magnetic resonance angiography (MRA): Demonstrates cerebral arterial or venous circulation and likely to replace conventional contrast angiography in some situations.

Arteriography is useful in evaluation of aneurysms and arteriovenous malformations.

MYELOGRAPHY

Since the introduction of MRI, this investigation is now needed infrequently, mainly in patients for whom MRI is contraindicated. Water-soluble contrast medium is introduced into the theca usually by means of a lumbar puncture. Views of the lumbar theca in lateral, anteroposterior and oblique projections demonstrate the spinal cord and nerve roots.

NORMAL BRAIN CT

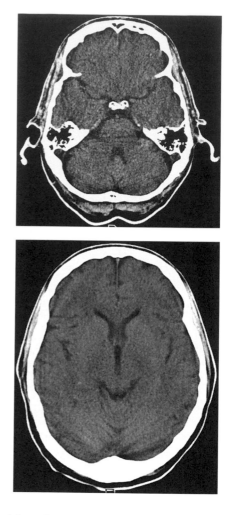

Fig. 10.2 Sections through a normal brain CT.

Each brain study of approximately 14 sections requires careful analysis but with practice it should be possible to spot major abnormalities at a glance. Compare the two sides with each other while looking through the series paying special attention to:

- midline shift;
- localized area of altered density;
- presence of mass lesion.

Cerebrospinal fluid appears black. Recent haemorrhage and haematoma appear white.

MRI OF NORMAL BRAIN

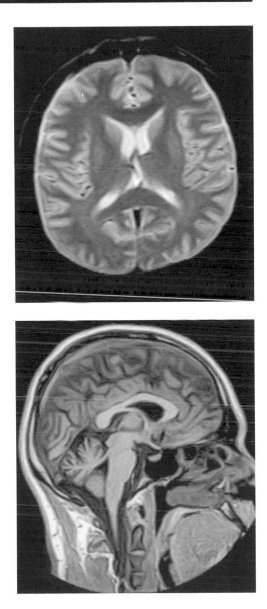

Fig. 10.3 Sections through a normal brain MR scan.

Instead of axial scanning in CT, two projections are usually utilized: axial and either coronal or sagittal. The appearances vary with the type of pulse sequence e.g. on T1 the CSF appears black (low signal) whereas on T2 it appears white (high signal). Both sequences are usually used for a study.

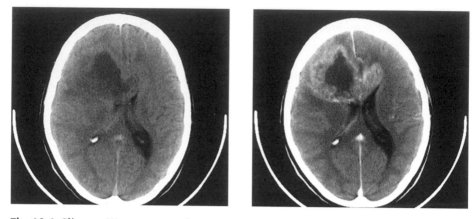

Fig. 10.4 Glioma: CT scan pre- and post-contrast showing a large frontal mass.

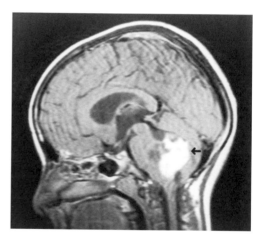

Fig. 10.5 Astrocytoma: coronal MRI in a child with a posterior fossa mass (arrow).

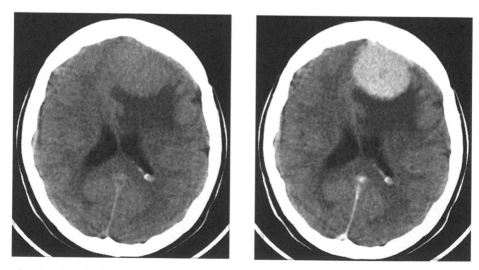

Fig. 10.6 Meningioma: CT scan pre- and post-contrast showing uniform enhancement.

PRIMARY INTRACRANIAL NEOPLASM

Primary brain tumours cause neurological symptoms due to distortion, pressure and displacement of adjacent structures. Even meningiomas or other benign tumours can cause a severe neurological deficit from the effect of expansion of the tumour in a confined space.

RADIOLOGICAL FEATURES

Generally, plain films are not contributory but may occasionally show calcification. Signs of raised intracranial pressure include dorsum sellae erosion, and in children sutural diastasis and cranial vault enlargement. MRI is the investigation of choice, but CT is still widely utilized due to its availability. For specific features, see below.

TYPES OF PRIMARY NEOPLASMS

Glioma. The commonest primary intracranial tumour and most frequent cause of pathological intracranial calcification; >50% of primary intracranial tumours are gliomas: astrocytoma, glioblastoma, oligodendroglioma and ependymoma. On CT, the tumour appears as an area of altered density, with surrounding oedema and mass effect. Significant enhancement usually follows intravenous contrast.

Meningioma. Meningiomas represent 15–20% of primary brain tumours. They are benign, well-defined lesions, arising from any part of the meningeal covering of the brain, frequent sites being the falx, parasagittal region, sphenoid wing and the convexity of the hemispheres. CT or MRI show well-defined lesions enhancing strongly and diffusely after intravenous contrast.

Acoustic neuroma. Arise in or near the Internal auditory canal, and may feature widening and erosion of the canal. MRI is more sensitive than CT in its detection.

Pituitary tumour. Plain films may show pituitary fossa enlargement or erosion. However, tumours such as prolactinomas are usually <1 cm in diameter and CT or preferably MRI is required for diagnosis.

Cerebellar tumour. The majority of intracranial tumours in children occur below the tentorium cerebelli: medulloblastoma is the most common intracranial tumour with ependymoma the next most frequent.

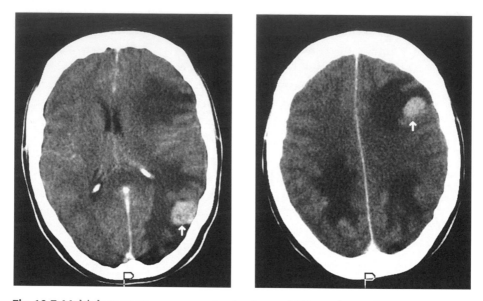

Fig. 10.7 Multiple metastases on a contrast enhanced CT scan (arrows).

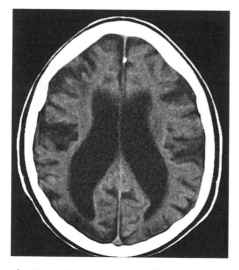

Fig. 10.8 CT scan in generalized cerebral atrophy with enlarged sulci and ventricles.

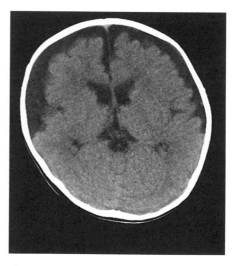

Fig. 10.9 CT scan of localized frontal cerebral atrophy in a child.

CEREBRAL METASTASES

Metastases are some of the commonest malignant cerebral lesions, involve any part of the brain and may be single or multiple. CT or MRI often cannot reliably distinguish between a primary neoplasm or a solitary secondary tumour, but the clinical setting may help. Multiple lesions are almost certainly metastases. Secondaries to the brain are commonly from bronchial, breast and gastrointestinal neoplasms.

RADIOLOGICAL FEATURES

Metastases can be haemorrhagic, cystic or calcified and they may cavitate; surrounding oedema is invariably present. After intravenous contrast, CT almost always shows enhancement of either the whole lesion or around the periphery, due to breakdown of the blood–brain barrier.

TREATMENT

- Palliative:
    dexamethasone reduces oedema and relieves headache; radiotherapy.
- Surgical resection occasionally for a solitary metastasis.

CEREBRAL ATROPHY

Atrophic changes in the brain are usually idiopathic. Causes include:
- degenerative conditions;
- trauma;
- drugs;
- infection (end stage);
- congenital conditions.

Correlation between atrophic changes and clinical features is poor.

RADIOLOGICAL FEATURES

- Irreversible loss of brain substance results in enlargement of the CSF spaces: the ventricles, basal cisterns, cerebral and cerebellar sulci. Ventricular dilatation may also be noted in hydrocephalus. However, in hydrocephalus, the ventricles dilate with relatively normal sulci whereas in atrophy there is usually both ventricular and sulcal enlargement.
- *Alzheimer's disease*: usually diffuse atrophy with relative sparing of cerebellum; the temporal lobes may be severely affected.
- *Pick's disease*: circumscribed lobar atrophy.
- *Other dementias*: usually non-specific diffuse atrophy as in Alzheimer's disease.

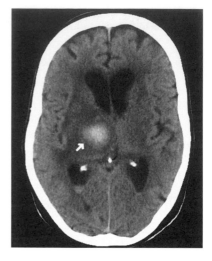

Fig. 10.10 CT scan: haemorrhagic middle-cerebral artery infarct (arrow).

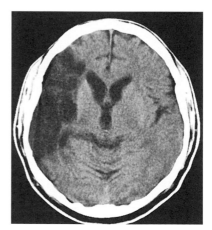

Fig. 10.11 CT scan: middle-cerebral artery infarct with extensive low density.

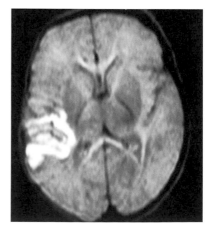

Fig. 10.12 MRI: left middle-cerebral artery infarct.

CEREBRAL INFARCT

Infarction of the brain results from a deficient cerebral circulation from thrombosis or an embolic event and clinically presents as a stroke. Predisposing factors include hypertension, diabetes, a family history and the many causes of atherosclerotic disease or emboli. Symptoms and signs vary depending on the site of infarction.

• A transient ischaemic attack (TIA) produces a focal neurological deficit in which complete recovery of function occurs within 24 hours.

• A stroke is one in which the neurological deficit persists.

• A lacunar infarct occurs as a result of occlusion of small intracerebral arteries.

RADIOLOGICAL INVESTIGATIONS

• CT/MRI of brain.

• Carotid artery imaging: magnetic resonance angiography (MRA)/Doppler ultrasound.

• Invasive arteriography should be avoided, but will occasionally be necessary.

RADIOLOGICAL FEATURES

The most useful role of CT/MRI is to confirm the presence of an infarct and to exclude haemorrhage or other abnormalities, thus expediting treatment with aspirin or anticoagulants.

• *CT:* may be and remain entirely normal, but most substantial infarcts that are going to be seen are visible within the first 24 hours. Initial abnormalities are often subtle. Loss of grey/white-matter differentiation evolves into reduced density, normally in an arterial supply territory, often with mild mass effect for the first few days and giving way to localized atrophic changes. About 15% develop haemorrhage, seen as an area of increased density.

• *MRI:* in association with MRA, is accurate and may demonstrate an occluded or stenosed vessel. The pattern and distribution of infarction is similar to CT.

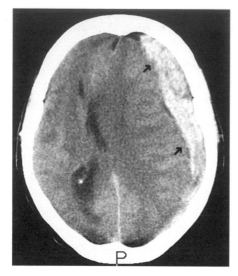

Fig. 10.13 CT brain: recent right subdural haematoma (arrows) with a significant midline shift.

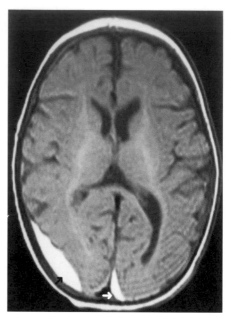

Fig. 10.14 MRI brain: subdural haematomas (arrows) in a 3-week-old infant.

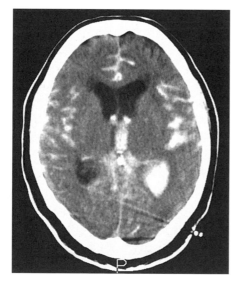

Fig. 10.15 CT brain: subarachnoid haemorrhage with blood in the sulci, third ventricle and the posterior horn of the left lateral ventricle.

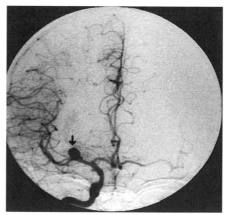

Fig. 10.16 Arteriogram: aneurysm of the right middle-cerebral artery (arrow).

EXTRACEREBRAL HAEMORRHAGE

Haemorrhage into the subdural or epidural space usually follows trauma. Neurological deterioration after a head injury should raise the suspicion of a haematoma whether or not there is a skull fracture. Chronic subdural haematoma may be found in the elderly, with blood accumulating slowly in the subdural space, possibly from a ruptured vein.

RADIOLOGICAL FEATURES

On CT, a subdural collection initially shows an area of peripherally placed crescentic fluid collection, lying adjacent to the cranial vault; it is seen as an area of altered density usually with a concave inner margin whereas an epidural haematoma has a convex inner border.

A recent haemorrhage is visualized as increased density (white) but subsequently this decreases to finally appear as an area of low density (black). Mass effect, with midline shift, indicates a significant subdural collection.

MRI is accurate for diagnosis and uses the same criteria as CT for differentiating a subdural from an epidural haematoma.

SUBARACHNOID HAEMORRHAGE

A subarachnoid haemorrhage is usually spontaneous, often the result of a ruptured aneurysm. Other causes include anticoagulant therapy and trauma. Sudden excruciating headache, nausea and vomiting, loss of conciousness or fits are the usual presenting symptoms. Hydrocephalus, either obstructive or communicating, is a recognized complication.

RADIOLOGICAL FEATURES

CT scanning is the investigation of choice, detecting recent haemorrhage more precisely than MRI. CT may show blood in the cisterns, fissures or ventricles. Arteriography is required in spontaneous subarachnoid haemorrhage to detect the source and site of bleeding, but should only be carried out if the patient is suitable for surgical intervention. Intracranial aneurysms are discovered in approximately 70% of cases. Unruptured aneurysms <4–5 mm are often not operated on unless shown to enlarge on interval imaging.

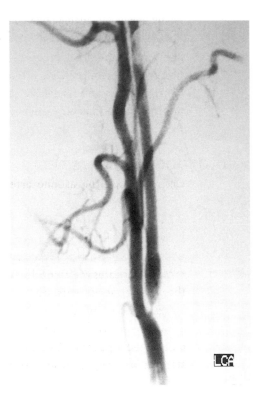

Fig. 10.17 Arteriogram demonstrating a critical stenosis at the origin of the left internal carotid artery.

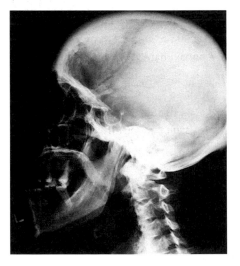

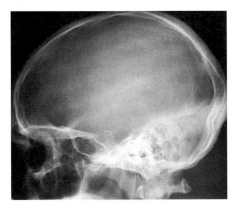

Fig. 10.18 Acromegaly with protruding mandible and enlarged pituitary fossa. Compare with the pituitary fossa of a normal lateral skull.

CAROTID ARTERY STENOSIS

Internal carotid artery stenosis may be either asymptomatic, present with transient ischaemic attacks (TIAs) or a stroke. In 30–40% of patients with TIAs, progression to a stroke results from distal infarction or embolization. The carotid artery may occlude totally without causing any symptoms.

RADIOLOGICAL INVESTIGATIONS

Colour Doppler ultrasound; arteriography.

RADIOLOGICAL FEATURES

• *Colour Doppler* accurately defines the stenosis, blood flow characteristics and alteration in peak velocities.
• *MRA* delineates the carotid arteries and any associated stenoses without the use of contrast material.
• *Arteriography*, either intravenous with computer subtraction or intra-arterial readily shows the anatomical abnormality, though the latter should be avoided if possible, because of the risk of serious complications. The stenosis is usually found at the origin of the internal carotid artery.

ACROMEGALY

Acromegaly results from an excessive secretion of growth hormone, usually from a pituitary adenoma. Approximately half the adenomas are < 1 cm in diameter.

RADIOLOGICAL INVESTIGATIONS

Plain films: lateral skull, hands and soft tissue of heel; MRI; CT.

RADIOLOGICAL FEATURES

MRI is the investigation of choice in order to demonstrate a pituitary adenoma.
A plain lateral skull may feature:
• enlarged pituitary fossa: late stages only;
• protruding mandible (prognathism);
• prominent sinuses.
Hands: become broad and spadelike.
Lateral heel: soft-tissue hypertrophy is best assessed by means of the heel pad thickness. In acromegaly, this is often >25 mm.
Joints: early degenerative arthritis.

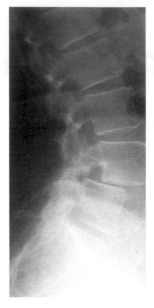
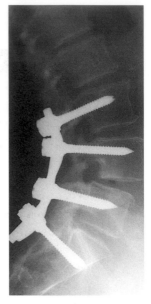

Fig. 10.19 Spondylolisthesis at L4/L5.

Fig. 10.20 Internal fixation to stabilize the abnormality.

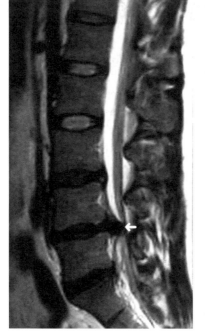
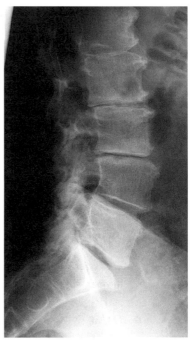

Fig. 10.21 MRI scan demonstrating a prolapsed disc at L4/L5 with posterior deviation of the theca (arrow).

Fig. 10.22 Typical degenerative changes in the lumbar spine with disc space narrowing.

SPONDYLOLISTHESIS

Spondylolisthesis refers to a slip of one vertebra on another, usually forwards but may occasionally be backwards. It may be degenerative (associated with severe osteoarthritis of the posterior facet joints, usually L4/L5), congenital, or posttraumatic, resulting in a defect in the pars interarticularis of the neural arch. It is often asymptomatic.

RADIOLOGICAL FEATURES

The slip is best demonstrated on a lateral projection of the lumbar spine and there may be an associated loss of disc space. The commonest affected levels are L4/L5 and L5/S1. CT/MRI evaluate the theca and any bony canal narrowing.

TREATMENT

- Conservative.
- Surgical: for a severe slip, internal fixation stabilizes the vertebra.

LUMBAR VERTEBRAL DISC PROLAPSE

Disc degeneration commonly occurs in the lower lumbar spine. Prolapse is due to extrusion of soft disc material from the nucleus pulposus and characterized by sciatic pain radiating from the buttock down the leg.
- L4/L5 prolapse (20% of cases): compression of the L5 root may result in foot drop and sensory loss of the outer aspect of the leg.
- L5/S1 prolapse (70% of cases): S1 root compression may cause an absent ankle jerk, with tingling and loss of sensation at the outer aspect of the foot.

RADIOLOGICAL FEATURES

- *Plain films.* Disc space narrowing, often with osteophyte formation, is best seen in the lateral projection.
- *CT.* Sensitive examination for posterior and lateral disc herniation in the lumbar spine. Demonstrates also hypertrophic degenerative changes in the facet joints which may cause bony canal stenosis.
- *MRI.* Distinguishes the nucleus pulposus from the annulus fibrosus with accurate diagnosis of degenerative discs. Degenerative disc disease is extremely common and must be correlated with clinical symptoms.
- *Myelography.* Injection of contrast into the spinal theca via a lumbar puncture, previously a common examination, but now almost obsolete.

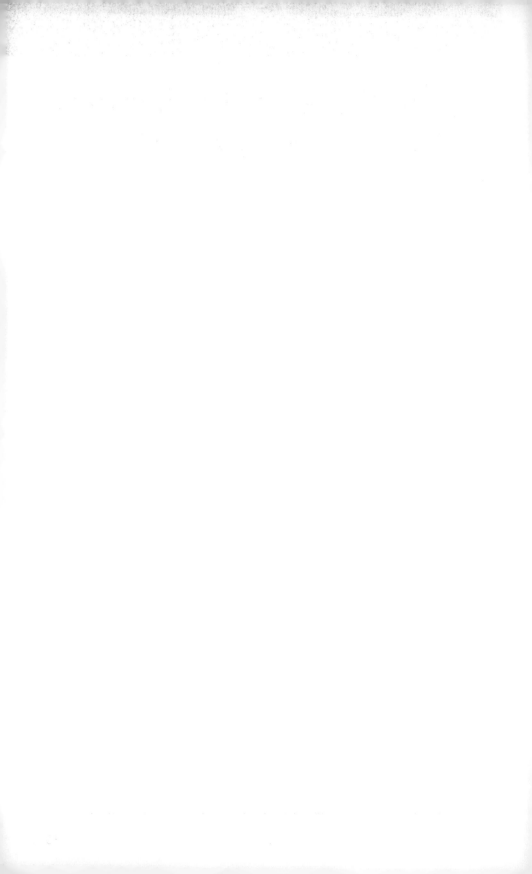

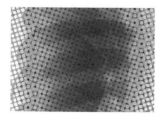

CHAPTER 11

Specific Radiological Investigations

RESPIRATORY TRACT

BRONCHIAL CARCINOMA

The majority of carcinomas are initially diagnosed by a chest X-ray. After a bronchoscopy is performed on a suspicious lesion, computed tomography (CT) or magnetic resonance imaging (MRI) evaluate the mass and any associated mediastinal lymph-node enlargement to assess operability of the tumour. Small nodes, less than 1 cm in diameter, may be due to reactive hyperplasia rather than neoplastic infiltration. In peripheral lesions, a percutaneous lung biopsy is indicated if bronchoscopy is unable to yield a suitable specimen for histology.

MULTIPLE LUNG METASTASES

CT is considerably more accurate at detecting secondary deposits than a chest X-ray. CT is required only when patient management would be altered by lung metastases or when treatment is available for certain carcinomas in spite of lung deposits, for example renal tumours, testicular tumours or osteogenic saroma. When a chest X-ray already shows metastases, CT is of little additional benefit.

CARDIOVASCULAR SYSTEM

DEEP-VEIN THROMBOSIS

This is a common problem; diagnosis is by either Doppler ultrasound or venography. Doppler scanning is non-invasive and without radiation risks; difficulty may be encountered in large limbs with poor visualization of the calf veins. Venography is performed less often, and in the evaluation of deep-vein thrombosis, is best reserved for inadequate Doppler studies.

PULMONARY EMBOLUS

A plain chest film may be entirely normal or show some non-specific signs, such as a pleural effusion or linear atelectasis. Ventilation/perfusion scans are moderately accurate and the majority of cases are diagnosed by this study, but occasionally the invasive technique of pulmonary angiography is required, with contrast injection directly into the pulmonary arteries. Contrast enhanced spiral CT of the chest may be helpful.

AORTIC ANEURYSM

Ultrasound is simple and efficient at detecting and following-up abdominal aneurysms. CT/MRI is required for suspected aortic dissection or a leaking aortic aneurysm. Arteriography may determine the origin of the aneurysm and demonstrate the peripheral circulation. In the thorax, ultrasound is limited to evaluation of the aortic root; CT with contrast or MRI are indicated for diagnosis of dissecting thoracic aneurysms.

STROKE

CT scanning may be normal up to 24 hours after the event, unless there is a haemorrhagic component; this appears as an area of high density.

HYPERTENSION

Onset of hypertension at a young age needs further investigation to discover a potentially curable cause, such as adrenal tumour or renal artery stenosis. Intravenous urography (IVU), ultrasonography and isotope studies may all imply a renovascular cause, but anatomical visualization by angiography is the definitive investigation. Spiral CT and magnetic resonance angiography (MRA) are likely to play an increasingly important role.

GASTROINTESTINAL TRACT

DYSPHAGIA

A barium swallow is the investigation of choice and must be performed prior to endoscopy to avert the danger of perforation from conditions such as a pharyngeal pouch. A suspected leak or perforation is investigated by means of water-soluble contrast agents. In patients in whom aspiration is a possibility, gastrografin is contraindicated, as this particular contrast agent in the lungs can cause severe pulmonary oedema.

CHANGE IN BOWEL HABIT

Barium enema or colonoscopy: colonoscopy may prove difficult in a tortuous colon with multiple redundant loops. If a colonic carcinoma is discovered, abdominal CT will stage the tumour (para-aortic lymphadenopathy and liver metastases).

GASTROINTESTINAL BLEEDING

Acute bleeding. Isotope scans may detect bleeding rates as low as 0.1 ml/min. Arteriography is less sensitive, and requires at least 1 ml/min but it may locate the exact site of haemorrhage for infusion of vasoconstrictors or embolization. Further evaluation of the small and large bowel can be carried out either by barium studies of the small bowel or colonoscopy of the large bowel.

Chronic bleeding. Colonoscopy or barium studies. Arteriography has a low success rate in detecting lesions but may discover tumours or angiodysplasia. Rarely, bleeding may be from a Meckel's diverticulum, when an isotope scan may detect ectopic gastric mucosa.

ABDOMINAL MASS

Ultrasound will identify the cause of most abdominal masses, for example those in liver, pancreas, kidneys or pelvis. Bowel masses may be difficult to visualize and require barium studies. CT is useful for further evaluation of an abdominal mass.

BILIARY TRACT

JAUNDICE

Ultrasound readily distinguishes an obstructive from a non-obstructive pattern by virtue of biliary duct dilatation and often confirms the level of obstruction. Endoscopic retrograde cholangiopancreatography (ERCP) will locate the site and often the cause of obstruction; common bile duct calculi can be removed at the same time. If ERCP is not technically successful, a transhepatic cholangiogram will provide similar information on the state of the biliary system; CT may be necessary for a suspected pancreatic tumour. Magnetic resonance cholangiopancreatography (MRCP) is proving to be a successful imaging technique.

ACUTE PANCREATITIS

Ultrasound may show a pleural effusion, enlargement of the pancreas, gallstones, common bile duct dilatation and collections or pseudocysts. Bowel gas often precludes optimum visualization of the pancreas and CT is often required. Intravenous contrast enhancement detects necrotic non-viable areas of the pancreas.

CHRONIC PANCREATITIS

A plain abdominal film showing pancreatic calcification is virtually diagnostic of chronic pancreatitis. Calcification and abnormal glandular structure can be readily detected by ultrasound and CT. ERCP confirms the state of the main pancreatic duct and its radicles.

HEPATOSPLENOMEGALY

Good quality plain films may show enlargement of the soft-tissue shadows of the liver and spleen. Ultrasound, however, is the more appropriate investigation to confirm liver or splenic enlargement.

LIVER METASTASES

Ultrasound is probably the best initial investigation; it is valuable as a screening test for patients with neoplastic disease. CT or MRI will also accurately localize secondary deposits; arteriography is rarely necessary.

URINARY TRACT

HAEMATURIA

The principal initial investigations are ultrasound and IVU. Ultrasound visualizes renal tumours, renal calculi, bladder tumours and prostatic enlargement. IVU will give a clear overall outline of the urinary tract as well as being a crude indicator of renal function; it may discover lesions such as calyceal or ureteric tumours, congenital abnormalities, papillary necrosis and renal calculi. Bladder tumours may not be accurately delineated due to overlying bowel and gas. Cystoscopy must always be performed even when all radiological investigations are normal.

RENAL MASS

A mass lesion detected at intravenous urography by calyceal distortion or alteration in renal size is further evaluated by ultrasound. Ultrasound will readily identify the size, shape and nature of the renal mass; the vast majority are found to be simple cysts and appear as well-defined echo-free lesions. If a mass is found to be solid, CT may ascertain the nature of the mass and assess local and distant spread.

CHRONIC RENAL FAILURE

Intravenous urography is not contraindicated, however a lack of contrast uptake, even with a mildly elevated urea, produces a technically unsatisfactory examination with poor visualization of the calyceal pattern; occasionally lesions suggesting tuberculosis or papillary necrosis may be identified. Ultrasound is useful for obstruction, renal size and as an aid to renal biopsy.

URINARY-TRACT INFECTION

Urinary-tract infections are common in women. IVU may discover a cause, such as renal calculus or congenital abnormality. In males, even a single episode of infection requires further investigation. Ultrasound, micturating cystography and isotope studies are all utilized in children.

RENAL-TRACT OBSTRUCTION

Renal-tract obstruction can occur in any part of the urinary tract but commonly result from pelvi-ureteric junction obstruction, ureteric calculus or bladder outlet obstruction. Calyceal or renal pelvic dilatation are easily demonstrated on ultrasound, though ureteric dilatation is not seen until a late stage. The commonest clinical problem is a ureteric calculus and ultrasound may demonstrate pelvicalyceal dlatation, but will not determine the site of obstruction: intravenous urography is often required and will accurately locate the level of obstruction. Antegrade and retrograde pyelograms are seldom necessary.

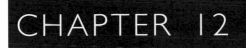

CHAPTER 12

Film-Viewing Hints

FILM-VIEWING HINTS

At some stage in your medical career, you will be asked for your opinion on a film, either in the final medical examination, ward rounds, conferences or postgraduate examinations. Efficient presentation of the film will create a good overall impression to an accompanying clinical case.

There is no substitute for having previously studied and analysed a large number of films, as a fairly substantial part of plain film and basic contrast radiology involves pattern recognition. There is no easy solution, and developing the ability to interpret them correctly is a long-term process. It is important, therefore, in your clinical years to be aware of the films that accompany patients and attempt to look at and analyse them, if necessary, in conjunction with the radiologist's report.

If you need some formal teaching sessions, persuade a radiologist to show you some common conditions. It is essential, however, that you request being taught on these, as the radiologist's collection will often be full of rare and obscure cases. You need to see cardiac failure, gallstones, pneumonia, etc. not Takayashu's arteritis, cysticercosis and aorto-enteric fistulae, however fascinating they may be.

The films in examinations are usually straightforward, dealing with common clinical problems. The majority are plain films, e.g. chest, abdomen, etc. Contrast examinations may include barium studies, intravenous urograms, biliary system, etc. When these are shown be aware that they can be reproduced in either a white format (used predominantly in this book) or one in which the contrast filled structures (arteries, veins, bladder, gut etc.) appear black. Ultrasound, computed tomography (CT) and magnetic resonance imaging (MRI) are more advanced investigations and only a rudimentary knowledge of these is required. You are unlikely to be asked about their interpretation, except for the very obvious, but should know where they fit in the sequence of investigating a patient, for example:
• jaundiced patient: ultrasound first, then endoscopic retrograde cholangiopancreatography (ERCP) or CT;
• lung mass: plain chest X-ray, bronchoscopy, CT/MRI, percutaneous lung biopsy.

Begin talking within 5–10 seconds of the film being displayed. Never stay silent for longer than 10 seconds. If you do not have a clue, start thinking aloud rather than keeping quiet. 'This is a chest X-ray and the lung fields appear clear. The cardiac shadow is normal in size and shape. Looking at the ribs . . . ' While you are describing this, you may come across an abnormal finding or if you are fortunate, the examiner may interrupt with a helpful suggestion. If you do see an abnormality, do not relax, but while talking about it, keep studying the film as there may be another one: for example, if there is a lung mass, there may be an associated rib metastasis or pleural effusion. One or two pertinent questions are permissible, but no more. Remember that the examiners are on your side and will try to be as helpful as they can.

When commenting on a film, take it in logical steps and do not jump from one to another. Complete each step and then progress to the next one.

- Identification of the film.
- Description of the abnormalities visible.
- Diagnosis or a differential diagnosis.

IDENTIFICATION OF THE FILM

Start by identifying the type of film presented to you. This might not be as simple as it seems. Plain films present no real problems but contrast exam-Inations may give rise to some difficulty.

The film may be approached In a technically correct manner: 'This is a chest X-ray taken in the posteroanterior projection. It is well penetrated and centred . . . ' However, this often produces a lengthy introduction and an acceptable alternative practice is to eliminate many of the preliminaries and proceed straight on to the film: 'This is a chest X-ray showing . . . ' or 'This is an abdominal X-ray showing . . . '

If a contrast examination is shown, of say, the bile ducts and you do not know whether it is a transhepatic, T-tube or a peroperative cholangiogram, a sensible approach to use would be to describe it initially as a contrast examination showing the bile ducts or similarly: 'This is a contrast examination showing the large bowel . . . ' or 'This is a contrast examination showing the bladder . . . ' and then later try to ascertain the exact nature of the investigation.

Make a quick mental note of the name If It is visible, as this may be important, first to distinguish between a male or female patient; second, to elucidate the ethnic origin, as both of these may give a clue to diagnosis. In the majority of cases, it is irrelevant, so do not pull the film off the viewing box or waste valuable time trying to find it. Do not point all over the film. If there is a particular area or abnormality that needs to be specified, identify it or point to it precisely, and then move away.

DESCRIPTION

This should be short and succinct. Avoid giving lengthy, verbose descriptions as the aim is to reach a conclusion. Concentrate on the major abnormality: in describing a chest X-ray with a lung mass, do not start talking about the heart size, ribs, etc. and leave the description of the mass to the last. The examiner may think that you have not seen it. Describe the mass first, and while you are doing this, look for any other abnormality. If none is seen, come to a diagnosis or a differential diagnosis.

Examiners will often give leading clues during the description, so take these gratefully. Remain calm and collected even when things are going badly. Whatever you do, do not disintegrate, no matter how badly you perceive the film viewing is going. If half-way through you realize that you are completely on the wrong track, or see something that contradicts your earlier description, do not struggle on. In this situation, it is reasonable to retract your statement and start all over again.

When viewing a film, for example a chest X-ray, you may need a lateral, or in the case of a contrast film, a control or preliminary film. Instead of asking 'Can I have a lateral,' it may be more appropriate to say 'Is a lateral of any help' or 'Is the plain film of any help.' The examiner will often reply that it is not, and you can proceed with the description. This is a minor point, but it all adds style towards the presentation.

DIAGNOSIS OR DIFFERENTIAL DIAGNOSIS

Only a few conditions will have a definitive or unequivocal diagnosis, for example pneumothorax or emphysema; most have a differential diagnosis. Remember the common conditions. It is important in a differential to mention the commonest disorders first and relegate the rarer ones to the bottom of the list. Neoplasm should head the list of a solitary lesion in the lung, not hamartoma or hydatid cyst.

Leave some room for manoeuvre, and unless you are sure, do not reach a definitive diagnosis as several answers are often possible. For example, a barium enema of ulcerative colitis can be described as having extensive ulceration in the colon, the appearances due to inflammatory bowel disease, most likely to be ulcerative colitis leaving enough manoeuvrability, in case it is Crohn's colitis.

TYPICAL EXAMPLES OF FILM DESCRIPTION

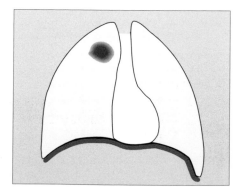

Fig. 12.1 Lung mass.

Lung mass

This is a chest X-ray showing a well defined opacity in the right upper zone. There is no calcification or cavitation associated with it. The appearances suggest a mass lesion and it is likely to be a neoplasm, either a primary or secondary. The differential diagnosis would also include other causes of a solitary lung opacity such as hamartoma, granuloma arteriovenous malformation, etc.

Cardiac enlargement, pericardial effusion

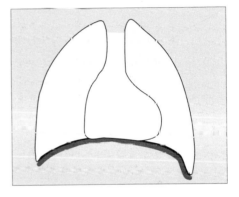

Fig. 12.2 Cardiac enlargement.

This is a chest X-ray showing a significantly enlarged cardiac shadow. The lungs show no abnormality. Causes of cardiomegaly would include cardiomyopathy, ischaemic heart disease or multiple valvular disease, but in view of the clear lung fields the possibility of a pericardial effusion should be considered. An ultrasound examination will confirm this.

Oesophageal stricture

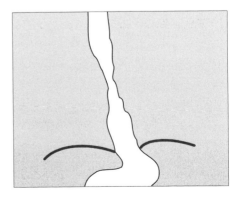

Fig. 12.3 Oesophageal stricture.

This examination is a barium swallow demonstrating narrowing in the lower oesophagus. There is mucosal irregularity associated with the narrowing and oesophageal carcinoma must be excluded. Secondary invasion from mediastinal tumours can also give rise to this appearance. The features are unlikely to be due to a benign stricture. An endoscopy with biopsy is necessary.

Gall stones

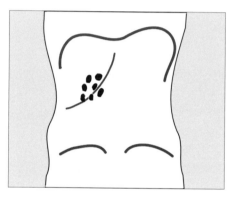

Fig. 12.4 Gall stones.

There are multiple opacities in the right hypochondrium on this plain abdominal film. These appear to be faceted and have the typical appearance of gall stones, but an ultrasound examination will readily confirm this.

Ureteric calculus

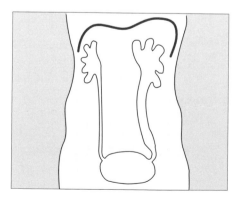

Fig. 12.5 Ureteric calculus.

The intravenous urogram shows distension of the left pelvicalyceal system. The ureter is dilated down to the level of the sacro-iliac joint and the appearances suggest obstruction. A pre-contrast film may demonstrate a calculus in this region.

Osteoarthritis

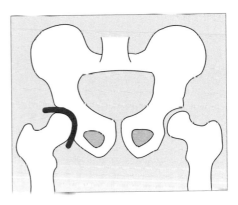

Fig. 12.6 Osteoarthritis.

This X-ray of the pelvis shows narrowing of the joint space at the right hip with osteophyte formation and articular irregularity. These are typical appearances of degenerative change.

Cerebral infarct

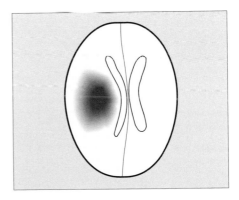

Fig. 12.7 Cerebral infarct.

This brain scan shows a low density area in the left parietal lobe. There is a slight mass effect with minor midline shift and compression of the left lateral ventricle. The appearances are likely to be due to a recent infarct in the middle cerebral artery territory.

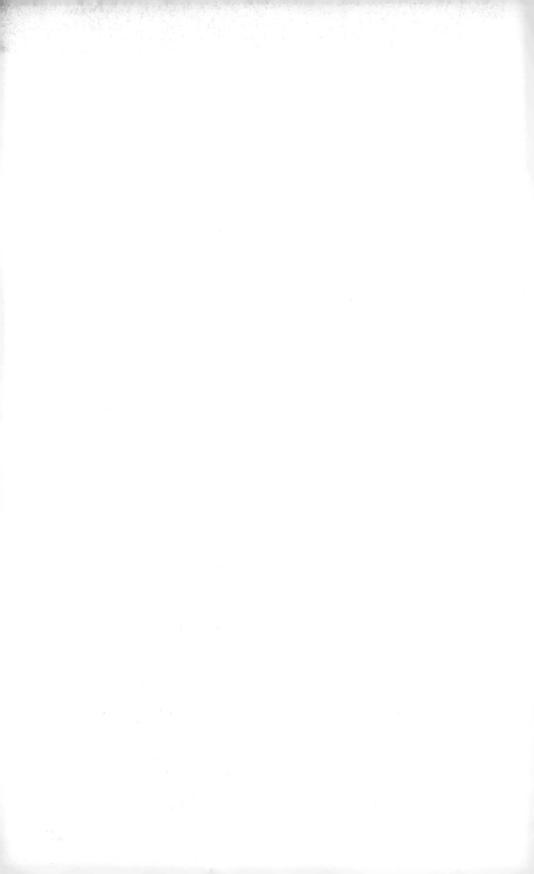

Index

The Lecture Notes Series

Bell et al
Tropical Medicine
4th edn

Blandy
Urology
5th edn

Bradley, Johnson &
Rubenstein
Molecular Medicine
1st edn

Bray et al
Human Physiology
3rd edn

Brewis
Respiratory Disease
4th edn

Bron, James & Chew
Ophthalmology
8th edn

Bull
**Diseases of the Ear,
Nose and Throat**
8th edn

Chamberlain & Malvern
Gynaecology
7th edn

Chamberlain
Obstetrics
7th edn

Coni, Davison & Webster
Geriatrics
5th edn

Duckworth
**Orthopaedics and
Fractures**
3rd edn

Elliott, Hastings &
Desselberger
Medical Microbiology
3rd edn

Ellis & Calne
General Surgery
8th edn

Farmer, Miller &
Lawrenson
**Epidemiology &
Public Health Medicine**
4th edn

Ginsberg
Neurology
1st edn

Graham Brown & Burns
Dermatology
7th edn

Gray et al
Cardiology
4th edn

Gwinnutt
Clinical Anaesthesia
1st edn

Hughes-Jones &
Wickramasinghe
Haematology
6th edn

Jeffcoate
Endocrinology
5th edn

Mandal, Wilkins, Dunbar &
Mayon-White
Infectious Diseases
5th edn

Moffat
Anatomy
2nd edn

Reeves & Todd
Immunology
3rd edn

Reid, Rubin & Whiting
Clinical Pharmacology
5th edn

Rubenstein, Wayne &
Bradley
Clinical Medicine
5th edn

Turner & Blackwood
Clinical Skills
3rd edn

Yates & Moulton
Emergency Medicine
2nd edn